THE INFANT-FEEDING TRIAD
Infant, Mother, and Household

Food and Nutrition in History and Anthropology
A series edited by John R. K. Robson, Medical University of South
Carolina, USA

Additional volumes in preparation

ISSN 0275-5769

THE INFANT-FEEDING TRIAD
Infant, Mother, and Household

BARRY M. POPKIN
University of North Carolina at Chapel Hill

TAMAR LASKY
Private Consultant

JUDITH LITVIN
University of Virginia

DEBORAH SPICER
New York State Department of Health

MONICA E. YAMAMOTO
University of Pittsburgh

Gordon and Breach Science Publishers

New York   London   Paris   Montreux   Tokyo

Gordon and Breach Science Publishers

Post Office Box 786
Cooper Station
New York, New York 10276
United States of America

Post Office Box 197
London WC2E 9PX
England

58, rue Lhomond
75005 Paris
France

Post Office Box 161
1820 Montreux 2
Switzerland

14-9 Okubo 3-chome
Shinjuku-ku, Tokyo 160
Japan

Library of Congress Cataloging-in-Publication Data

The Infant-feeding triad.

   (Food and nutrition in history and anthropology, ISSN 0275-5769; v. 5)
   Bibliography: p. 205
   Includes index.
   1. Infants—Nutrition.   2. Mothers—Nutrition.
3. Infants—Nutrition—Social aspects.   I. Popkin,
Barry M.   II. Series
RJ216.I498   1986   363.8'2   86-9870

CONTENTS

v

FIGURES

TABLES

PREFACE

Over the past few years a multidisciplinary group at the Carolina Population Center, University of North Carolina at Chapel Hill, has been doing research integrating social science and biomedical methodologies for the analysis of nutrition, health, and population topics. Focusing on analyses at the household and community levels, we have tried to understand the problems and constraints individuals and households face in attempting to meet their health and nutrition needs. A primary emphasis of the work has been developing methodologies for analyzing the patterns and determinants of breast-feeding and infant supplementary feeding in low-income countries and the United States.

We initially studied infant-feeding patterns and determinants not only because we believed that these were major nutrition policy topics of import for low-income countries, but also because we felt they comprised a topic area for which more rigorous research methodologies for analysis of population-based data were needed. In reviewing the research in this area, we found that, while the consequences of breast-feeding on infant morbidity have been extensively studied, little attention has been paid to the wide range of other ways breast-feeding affects the infant, mother, and household. Moreover, we found that very few scholars have attempted to understand how other types of infant foods affect the infant and others in the household.

This manuscript was originally prepared in 1981–82 and the information used in the design of a longitudinal infant-feeding study to investigate many of the unanswered questions. Other reviews by members of this group on women's nutrition (Hamilton *et al.*, 1984) and breast-feeding (Popkin *et al.*, 1982) have preceded this effort. Since 1982, two important sets of related literature reviews by other scientists have also been published. Staff of the National Institutes of Health, National Center for Health Statistics and Center for Disease Control, in several separate papers reviewed the effects of infant feeding on infant growth and morbidity, and relationships between infant feeding and fertility. These reviews were published in a supplement of *Pediatrics* in 1984 [vol. 74(4), part 2]. Another review by Feachem and Koblinsky (1984) related breast-feeding to diarrhea. In updating this manuscript we were able to use additional materials from these two efforts. We address numerous issues not covered in either of the publications above.

The Carolina Population Center (CPC) received a gift to assist this publication from the Nestlé's Coordinating Center for Nutrition Research, and our research group received an additional grant directly from the center. We thank Nestlé and CPC for their assistance.

From its inception, preparing this review has been a collaborative effort among its several authors. We have met often to clarify our focus and to ensure that we were addressing the key methodological issues. Although advice has come from various individuals, this book largely represents the views of its coauthors. Tamar Lasky had a role in conceptualizing the issues; she drafted the section on definitions of infant feeding and the epidemiological sections on infant growth and morbidity. Deborah Spicer drafted the chapters on maternal nutritional status, the household, the introduction, and the summary. In addition she coordinated the administrative aspects of the initial draft of the whole manuscript. Judith Litvin prepared the sections on immunological issues in infant morbidity, specific infant nutritional issues, and the interactions between infant growth and morbidity. Monica E. Yamamoto prepared the section on infant feeding and fecundity. I laid out the general framework and listed the specific issues and hypotheses to be addressed. I worked with each of the coauthors on their sections and coordinated the final preparation of the manuscript.

Lynn Igoe edited the manuscript and prepared many of the figures, with the help of Bayard Hollingsworth. Catheryn Brandon coordinated the word-processing staff and proofreaders, Ellen Payne, David Claris, and Jeff Slagle. Nancy Dole Runkle assisted with computerization. Annette Hedaya prepared the final copies of the Indexes. Final proofreading was in the capable hands of Margaret E. Morse, Margaret C. McGinty, and Margaret Mauney, who took care of many other details. All are staff members of the Carolina Population Center. We are grateful to Eilene Z. Bisgrove, a doctoral student in nutrition at the University of North Carolina at Chapel Hill, for creating the cover illustration.

We thank John Akin, John Briscoe, and Meg McCann, all of the University of North Carolina at Chapel Hill; Thad Jackson, formerly vice-president, Nestlé's Coordinating Center for Nutrition, Inc.; and an anonymous reviewer for their contributions in reviewing specific sections. We are grateful to Abraham Horwitz and Michael C. Latham for their advice during the early stages of thought on this book. Dr. Horwitz is director emeritus, Pan American Health Organization, and chairman, International Nutrition Committee, National Academy of Science, and a member of the United Nations Coordinating Committee on Nutrition. Dr.Latham is professor of international nutrition, Cornell University. We also thank Dr. John R. K. Robson, editor of this series of books for Gordon and Breach, for his assistance in bringing this publication to fruition.

Barry M. Popkin

ABOUT THE AUTHORS

BARRY M. POPKIN, Professor of Nutrition in the School of Public Health at the University of North Carolina at Chapel Hill, has been involved in integrating socioeconomic and biomedical issues in research in the nutrition field for over 15 years. He has been actively involved in a large number of research and policy activities related to infant and maternal nutrition in both the United States and low-income countries. He received his undergraduate training from the University of Wisconsin and the University of New Delhi and graduate training from the Universities of Pennsylvania and Wisconsin and Cornell University. He earned a doctorate in agricultural economics from Cornell. Before his association with the University of North Carolina, Popkin was a special field staff member of the Rockefeller Foundation stationed in the Philippines, associate director of the International Nutrition Program of Cornell University, and a research associate of the Institute for Research on Poverty, the University of Wisconsin.

TAMAR LASKY, an epidemiologist, has done research in the areas of reproductive health and maternal and child health. Her undergraduate degree was in Biology from Grinnell College and her doctoral degree is in Epidemiology from the School of Public Health at the University of North Carolina at Chapel Hill. She has research experience at the University of North Carolina at Chapel Hill, and before that, at Cornell University Medical School and the Population Council. At present she is living in Baltimore and doing consulting work.

JUDITH LITVIN, presently postdoctoral fellow in Anatomy and Cell Biology at the University of Virginia, has spent her research efforts on issues of embryonic development. She received her undergraduate degree from Queens College in New York and her graduate training at the University of North Carolina at Chapel Hill. Prior to her graduate training she was employed as a research assistant at Harvard University in the field of immunochemistry.

DEBORAH SPICER has a bachelor's degree from Brown University and an MPH in Nutrition from the University of North Carolina at Chapel Hill. She has been involved in research on issues related to maternal and infant nutrition. She is currently with the New York State Department of Health.

ABOUT THE AUTHORS

MONICA E. YAMAMOTO, a nutrition epidemiologist, is currently a research fellow in cardiovascular epidemiology at the University of Pittsburgh. She has worked in applied public health nutrition and nutrition research for the past 20 years, including seven years as a consultant with the Taiwan and Philippine national family planning and nutrition programs. Her research work has focused on international and national maternal and child nutrition issues. She received her undergraduate training at Immaculate Heart College in Los Angeles; her clinical nutrition training at the Peter Bent Brigham Hospital in Boston; and her graduate training at the University of California at Berkeley, the University of the Philippines, the University of North Carolina at Chapel Hill, and the University of Pittsburgh.

1
INTRODUCTION

Today, in low-income countries, although the vast majority of women still initiate breast-feeding, important changes are occurring in breast-feeding patterns. A wide variety of other foods are being fed to the infant at an earlier age. Full or partial breast-feeding continues to be almost universal during the first six months of life in most countries in Asia and Africa. In only a few countries is there evidence of a decline in the proportion of children ever breast-fed. However, a general decline in breast-feeding duration, especially in Latin America, and an earlier introduction of other infant foods appear to be occurring in most regions of the world (Ferry, 1981; Notzon, 1984; Popkin et al., 1982). The exact nature of the changes in overall infant-feeding patterns is not clear from available publications. Nevertheless, changes in infant-feeding practices have led to growing concern about their implications, reflected in part by the controversy surrounding the promotion and use of commercially prepared infant formulas.

We feel that the current controversy surrounding the impact of changes in infant-feeding patterns is limited in several respects. First, most literature on feeding-pattern choices has focused on effects of breast-feeding or bottle-feeding on infant growth and morbidity. Such a focus produces an unbalanced picture ignoring effects on mother and household. Second, dialogue and policy recommendations have focused on differences in effects between breast milk and commercial infant formula and have overlooked infants in low-income countries who, if not wholly breast-fed, are being given a wide variety of other foods—including evaporated, condensed sweetened, and skim milk, undiluted animal milks, and gruels, as well as various kinds of commercial formulas. Third, research on the impacts of different feeding methods has not usually been designed to investigate the mechanisms underlying these impacts. For instance, feeding affects infant health through three intervening pathways—its exposure to pathogens, nutritional status, and immune status. The relative contribution of each pathway to morbidity is not understood. Therefore, only limited policy analysis is possible from most available studies.

Each of these unexplored issues is important for the development and implementation of policies to promote health and economic development. The major purpose of this book is to broaden the scope of discussion of the effects of infant feeding by considering aspects of the infant-feeding controversy in some depth. Emphasis will be on developing hypotheses to be tested in future studies and on identifying methodological problems inherent in such studies.

Infant feeding is not simply a biological process in response to the metabolic demands of a baby. It is also a complex web of behaviors involving actions and reactions of other people. Full analysis of the effects of a particular infant-feeding regimen must investigate the effects of feeding on the mother and household as well as on the infant. Figure I-1 shows how an infant-feeding pattern is likely to affect directly not only infant nutritional status, growth, and morbidity, but also the mother's nutritional status and fertility and the household's use of time and money. The primary effects of infant feeding on each immediate participant—infant, mother, other household members—are also likely to produce secondary effects on each other. Because many of these effects occur simultaneously, it is difficult to distinguish between them. What is usually measured is the net effect of infant feeding on any one outcome. It is not always easy to determine what portion of the net effect is because of direct (primary) effect of infant feeding on that outcome and what is due to an indirect (secondary) impact operating through effects on other outcomes. For example, breast-feeding may directly affect infant morbidity by providing immunologic elements to the infant. Lactation may also make nutrient demands on a mother which her dietary intake and nutrient stores cannot

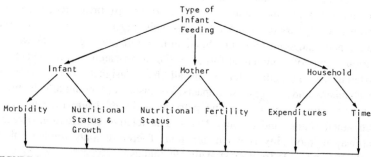

FIGURE I-1   Effects of infant feeding.

meet. Maternal physiologic adjustments may occur resulting in a decrease in breast milk production that may have a secondary effect on infant morbidity through a reduction in its nutritional status. What is usually measured is the child's total morbidity experience. Without further investigation of the interactions among maternal nutritional status, breast milk production, and infant nutritional status, it is not clear which pathway is the major contributor to infant morbidity.

Besides being limited to studying the effects of infant feeding on the infant itself, previous research has not always been clear about other foods to which breast milk was being compared. Different foods could have dramatically different impacts on the outcomes of interest. For instance, there may be significant differences in growth between breast-fed infants and those fed watery gruels, but there is less evidence of significant differences in growth between breast-fed infants and those fed properly prepared commercial formulas. We attempt to clarify this situation by considering two separate hypotheses. In the first, we contrast breast-feeding with all other feeding practices with respect to the dependent variables (infant growth, morbidity, maternal nutritional status, etc.). In the second hypothesis, we contrast other infant foods with each other and consider possible effects on the same dependent variables.

The first hypothesis has been the focus of most research, although previous studies have rarely identified what kinds of foods the nonbreast-fed or never-breast-fed infants received. To review and draw conclusions from these studies, it is necessary to use the first hypothesis as an organizing theme. Comparing breast milk and other foods also makes inherent sense since breast milk has distinct qualities that set it apart from all other foods. For example, a great deal of evidence suggests unique immunological properties of breast milk. No evidence suggests that other foods vary in their effect on the infant's immune status. Thus the chapter on morbidity focuses on the hypothesis that the infant's risk of infectious disease varies with the level of breast-feeding. Again, there is evidence that breast-feeding may affect fecundity and no evidence to suggest that other infant foods affect it; chapter 8 thus focuses on the hypothesis that fecundity levels increase with decreasing levels of breast-feeding.

The second hypothesis goes beyond what has been done in the past to consider the differential effects of feeding various kinds of food other than breast milk. Many more research gaps exist with respect to this latter hypothesis. While the breast-feeding/other foods contrast has the greatest implications for infant morbidity and mortality, maternal fecundity, and time allocation, as the infant grows and more foods are introduced in its diet, the varying effects of other foods become of increasing interest. Various categories of other infant food will require different levels of expenditures, skills, preparation and feeding time, and also carry different levels and types of pathogens and nutrients. These other foods are crucial not only for supplementing breast-feeding but for feeding infants who have never been breast-fed and those who have been completely weaned from the breast.

Studying the consequences of different infant-feeding methods is not merely academic. Identifying effects of various infant-feeding routines is essential for the formation of health and development policies. Policy decisions in several areas can affect the health and economic well-being of infants, mothers, and household members by influencing the choice of infant-feeding method. Policy decisions guide the training of health professionals on the subject of infant feeding and determine educational messages directed to the public at large. Policy also determines what types of infant foods are made available in supplemental feeding programs, the ages of infants eligible for such programs, the foods supported by price subsidies, and postpartum maternal labor policies. To make wise decisions about these policies, planners need accurate, clear, and complete information on consequences of various infant-feeding patterns.

Many different issues must be considered when trying to determine the overall effect of infant-feeding patterns on any outcome. Issues include change in effect with the infant's age and persistence of an effect after stopping a particular type of feeding. Knowledge of each issue is necessary for formation of appropriate policies. Because these issues have not been dealt with comprehensively in the literature, we describe some of the more important ones. Each is examined thoroughly throughout this book.

First, effects of an infant-feeding method may vary with age. Thus, policy concerning infant feeding needs to be age specific. Not only do an infant's nutritional needs vary with age, but so does its vulnerability to changes in feeding pattern. A three-week-old infant may suffer from being weaned completely from breast milk. The same process may not affect a nine-month-old infant so strongly. As an infant's nutritional needs increase with age, the mother may be unable to meet them without sacrificing her own nutritional health. The time inputs needed by the feeding process also change with the infant's age. For a young infant with an immature immunologic system any food other than breast milk needs to be carefully prepared to avoid contamination. An older infant may be able to tolerate a more contaminated, less time-intensive food.

Second, policy affecting infant-feeding choices needs to be based not only on effects at different infant ages, but also on the accumulation of effects over time. These two viewpoints may lead to different conclusions about the effects of different feeding practices. For instance, while the growth rate of a wholly breast-fed infant 12 months of age may be less than that of an infant fed other foods, the accumulated growth rate over the 12-month period may be higher for the breast-fed infant. Similarly, time inputs by the mother and other household members to the feeding process may be greater for a 12-month-old breast-fed infant than for a 12-month-old infant who feeds itself from food prepared for the rest of the household. The accumulation of time spent over the 12-month period, however, may be less in the case of the breast-fed infant. Recommendations need to be based on information from both viewpoints.

Third, feeding special foods to infants takes place during a relatively short portion of the human life span, but because of the many growth and developmental processes occurring during that time, feeding may affect many aspects of later life. This fact, too, is important to the development of policy recommendations. Infant feeding must be looked at in a broader context. Information must be obtained on the persistence of the effects of feeding methods once the particular method has been discontinued. For example, a difference in morbidity experience may be found at 3 months of age between breast-fed infants and those fed other foods, but there may not be any difference in morbidity at 18 months when both infants are eating similar, adult foods. Similarly, a woman's nutritional status may decline while she is breast-feeding, but after lactation ceases, she may be able to replenish her stores and return to her prepregnant nutritional status.

Fourth, information on the effects of exclusive breast-feeding or feeding exclusively with other foods is of limited usefulness. Mixed-feeding may be the more common practice in many cultures and it may be the optimal type of infant feeding, especially for older infants. Knowledge of the type of relationship between the proportion of an infant's intake from various food sources and the level of effect, be it on infant growth and morbidity or other outcomes, becomes important for the development of appropriate recommendations. The relationship between infant growth and the percentage of intake from breast milk may be varied, for example, direct, linear, and continuous, suggesting that each incremental increase in contribution of breast milk will bring about an equal incremental increase in growth, with optimal growth being achieved at 100 percent breast-feeding. Or the relationship may be discontinuous, with a peak in growth at some combination of breast-feeding and feeding other foods, beyond which the growth rate may decline. In the latter case, increasing the contribution of breast-feeding beyond the threshold point may negatively affect the infant, and the appropriate policy would be to recommend mixed-feeding.

Fifth, policy decisions should be based, as much as possible, on the summation of effects on different outcomes. Developing policies based on the effects of infant-feeding methods on an isolated outcome is inappropriate and may be detrimental in a broader context. For example, while the breast-fed infant may be better off in terms of lower morbidity than its counterpart given other foods, the breast-feeding mother may experience a decline in her nutritional status compared with the nonbreast-feeding mother. Thus policy based solely on effects on the infant may be detrimental to the mother. Similarly, while the nonbreast-feeding mother may have a higher nutritional status than her breast-feeding counterpart, other members of the former's household may experience a decrease in their food allotment because of the cost of purchasing foods for the infant. It is difficult to express these different outcomes in terms of one common denominator so that the effects on one outcome can be directly compared with the effects on other outcomes. At some point, a subjective decision has to be made. At the least, policy makers need to be aware of the multiplicity of outcomes and trade-offs between them.

Finally, it is important to understand the interactions between outcomes, that is, how one outcome may affect others. Policy designed to have an impact on one particular outcome may have far-reaching consequences which should be considered in advance of implementation. For example, breast-feeding places a heavy demand on the mother's nutritional status. The mother may respond to this increased demand by lowering her physical activity, such as decreasing her wage-earning activities, thus affecting household income. Or, her production of breast milk may suffer. Feeding an infant with foods other than breast milk may involve additional costs to the household, but the household may compensate by decreasing expenditures on other items or by reallocating the time of some of its members toward more income-generating activities. Any attempt to direct policy on the basis of an evaluation of the effects of different feeding methods must consider the means and extent of compensation and reallocation which occur with individuals and within households.

Although in this book the scope of the discussion of the consequences of infant feeding is considerably broadened, it is not all-encompassing and, because of time limitations, some issues are not covered sufficiently. This book focuses on the short-term effects of infant feeding, limiting the period under consideration to the first two years of life, with a strong emphasis on the first year. We do not review the effects of infant feeding on later development of chronic diseases and on important issues in child development such as maternal-infant bonding and social and intellectual development, or the effects of feeding method on speech development. While these issues are important, it is felt that in Third World populations, the issues of infant growth and morbidity are significantly more crucial. This book is also limited to a review of micro-level effects of infant feeding—effects on individuals and households. Effects of infant feeding on macro-level concerns such as gross national product and foreign exchange are not discussed.

A major issue beyond the scope of this book concerns the effects of infant feeding on low-birth-weight (LBW) infants (weighing less than 2500 g), both preterm and small for gestational age (SGA). Although statistics on rates of low birth weight in low-income countries are not routinely collected and published, surveys in individual countries indicate the problem is significant. One review calculated that the global LBW rate (including high- and low-income countries) was approximately 16 percent of live births (Petros-Barvazian and Behar, 1979). This review further calculated that 80 percent of LBW infants in low-income countries were small, full-term infants rather than preterm infants. Another review found the proportion ranged from 4.1 percent of live births in Sweden to 45 percent in India. India, Burma, Singapore, and Papua, New Guinea, had rates greater than 20 percent (Boldman and Reed, 1976; WHO, 1980, 1984).

Current research indicates that LBW infants differ from their full-sized, full-term counterparts in several ways which may alter the effect of different feeding methods on a variety of outcomes. The LBW infant is likely to be less mature immunologically (see chapter 4). Because of the immunologic properties of breast milk, and the heightened possibility of contamination by use of foods other than breast milk, the effects of type of feeding on morbidity of LBW infants may be more pronounced than that of normal infants.

Immaturity in other organs and biochemical systems contributes to differing nutritional requirements of LBW infants. For instance, fat absorption is lower in preterm infants (AAP, 1977; Battaglia and Simmons, 1978; CPS, 1981; Hamosh et al., 1978) and LBW infants suffer from an inability to metabolize certain amino acids (AAP, 1977; CPS, 1981). The ideal growth rate for preterm (but not SGA) infants is generally considered equivalent to comparable intrauterine growth rates (although this is somewhat controversial), which is higher than the normal postnatal growth rate. This higher growth rate results in higher nutrient requirements, especially for protein and calcium (AAP, 1977; Battaglia and Simmons, 1978; Brandt, 1978; Fomon *et al.*, 1977). Finally, LBW infants often have lower than normal stores of some nutrients, including essential fatty acids and iron (AAP, 1977; CPS, 1981; Seip and Halvorsen, 1956).

These differences in nutrient needs of LBW infants are reflected in differences in the breast milk their mothers produced. These mothers appear to be able to produce adequate *quantities* of milk (CPS, 1981). The *quality* of their milk seems to differ in several respects, including increased protein and calcium content, and may be biologically tailored to the special needs of their infants (AAP, 1985; Atkinson *et al.*, 1978, 1980; S. J. Gross *et al.*, 1980). In addition to differences in nutritional needs, LBW infants may require greater inputs of time from the mother and other household members than do normal weight infants.

Because they make up a significant proportion of the infant population in low-income countries, the effects of feeding methods on LBW infants need to be studied. However, because of their unique needs, LBW infants need to be studied as a separate group.

In chapter 2 we discuss general issues concerning use of infant feeding as an independent variable and the methodological implications of various categorization schemes. We also present definitions being used in this book. The remainder of the book examines a series of dependent (or outcome) variables considered to be possible consequences of infant-feeding practices. In chapters 3, 4, and 5 we look at feeding effects on infant morbidity, mortality, and growth. In chapter 6 we assess the impact of infant feeding on infant health. In chapters 7 and 8 we consider effects on the mother, including nutritional status and fecundity, and in chapter 9 we examine effects on the household such as time allocation and expenditures. In each chapter we discuss the relationship between infant-feeding practices and the dependent variable, theoretical and epidemiological evidence for hypotheses about these relationships, and methodological issues involved in testing these hypotheses. We are particularly concerned with evaluating studies with respect to their design, choice of study populations, analytical techniques, and how they handle issues of confounding variables. These discussions of methodological issues lead to suggestions for further research, improvements in research design, and the formation of hypotheses which need further testing.

2

DEFINING INFANT-FEEDING PRACTICES

In using infant feeding as an independent variable, one may consider the effects that exposure to a certain feeding regimen may have on several outcomes: morbidity, mortality, growth, emotional and physical development, maternal endocrine status, maternal reproductive potential, mother-infant bonding, or various social and economic factors. Defining these feeding regimens and categorizing infants into feeding groups depends on (1) the outcomes to be examined and the hypotheses being tested, which are based on a theoretical body of evidence, and (2) practical considerations of the feasibility of collecting the data of interest and the desire to set up categories with adequate numbers of subjects. Because theoretical vantage points and practical considerations vary from setting to setting, infant-feeding practices are defined differently in different studies, limiting the comparability of study results.

THEORETICAL CONSIDERATIONS

Since infant-feeding practices are postulated to have a variety of effects on the infant, mother, and household, it may be difficult to devise a categorization scheme to encompass every theoretical viewpoint. From a nutritional point of view, there may be a desire to consider the proportion of calories, proteins and lipids, and other essential nutrients derived from a particular food source and the change in proportion over time postpartum. From an immunological viewpoint, considering the introduction of pathogens or the absolute quantity of immunoglobulins ingested may be desirable. In terms of maternal reproductive function, information on duration, frequency, timing, and intensity of suckling would be valuable. When considering what behaviors lead to prolonged and more complete breast-feeding, the relationship between overall breast-feeding duration, frequency of feedings in a day, cues leading to breast-feedings, patterns of night feedings, and number, pattern, and type of supplementary feedings should be examined. Finally, behavioralists may be most interested in the nature of the mother-infant interaction during a feeding, and its effect on the child's personality development.

Thus a variety of characteristics should be included when describing a particular feeding, a feeding pattern within a 24-hour period, or changes in feeding patterns that occur as the infant grows. One or more of the characteristics in table II-1 may need to be considered. A study could describe infant-feeding practices within a given 24-hour period and over time as the infant grows. The researcher would want to know the frequency of a particular type of feeding in a 24-hour period, and the change in feeding patterns with the infant's age. Such data would not be relevant to every research project; they are difficult to collect accurately, since feeding patterns vary tremendously from day to day, and over the first year of the infant's life. Infant-feeding practices may be described by a series of multidimensional continuums for many of the above characteristics, varying within an age group, across cultures, social classes, and other socioeconomic variables, and within a cultural or social group over time, changing as the infant grows. Placing infants in two, three, or four categories will obscure much of the variation when several specific hypotheses are tested. In evaluating the research it is important to ask whether the categorization scheme used is appropriate to the hypotheses being tested, results in appropriate methods of statistical analysis, and makes maximal use of the data collected.

TABLE II-1

Characteristics of an individual infant feeding

Content (breast milk, other milk, other foods)
Food source (breast, commercial, home-grown, home-prepared)
Food storage (none needed, sealed containers, refrigerator, none used)
Quantity of particular food fed to infant
Mode of feeding (breast, bottle, cup, spoon, hand, other utensil)
Duration of feeding
Who feeds infant
Caretaker-infant interaction at feeding
Cues eliciting feeding
Night feedings (frequency, patterns)
Intensity of suckling, emptying of breast

PRACTICAL CONSIDERATIONS

Collecting Infant-Feeding Data: Measurement Issues

Realities of data collection limit the information available to the researcher, and in turn influence the categorization scheme. Individual infant-feeding practices may be determined from medical records (records of maternity stay, pediatric or well-baby records) or from the mother herself. Each data source has advantages and disadvantages that limit the data that can be collected. The value of medical records varies with the health care system and how a given population uses it. Where health care use is widespread and uniform, medical records can provide consistent, prospectively collected data on feeding practices on large sample sizes of a given population. These data will probably be limited to dates when various feeding regimens begin and end—and problems encountered with them.

Information can be collected from mothers in various ways. Recall data, an interview, or questionnaire asking a mother to describe how her baby was fed prior to the date of data collection will vary in accuracy with the time interval involved, the level of detail requested, and the mother's sociodemographic characteristics. The researcher may thus be able to reach a population that does not use the health care system, or one with access to widely differing qualities of health care, but the information obtained will be dates when various feeding regimens began and ended, with perhaps some of the items in table II-1 concerning current feeding status.

To gather the type of the information table II-1 suggests, the researcher could prospectively follow a group of mothers with telephone or home interviews, have them record daily feeding data, or visit the home regularly for actual observation. The more intensive the data collection, the greater the imposition on the mother, and the more likely that (1) the cost of the study will increase; (2) mothers will refuse to participate; and (3) the intense observation will alter mothers' behaviors. Thus, practical constraints of data collection must be balanced against theoretical considerations.

Sample Size Issues

The need for adequate sample sizes in each category may result in categories which disregard theoretical divisions. In modern industrialized settings it is often difficult to find adequate numbers of the exclusively breast-fed; instead a category called "essentially" or "primarily" breast-fed is often used. Similarly, in non-Western settings it may be difficult to find adequate numbers of exclusively bottle-fed (absolutely no breast-feeding) babies, and they may be combined with the partially breast-fed. These categorization schemes, while convenient, may weaken the researcher's ability to test a particular hypothesis and may obscure dose-response or threshold relationships.

CATEGORIZATION AND ANALYTICAL METHODS

Depending on the hypothesis being tested and available data, it may be advisable to avoid categorization and treat infant-feeding practices as continuous variables. Life table and related multivariate analyses are suited to examining (1) duration of a particular feeding regimen; (2) onset of a particular outcome (menstruation, illness of child, weaning, or any other time-dependent event); and (3) comparison across groups (sociodemographic, medical, groups in particular health programs, or groups categorized by degree of supplementation, frequency of suckling, or other variable hypothesized to be associated with the outcome variable). Such analyses are appropriate when feeding practices are independent or dependent variables. They allow consideration of duration, separated from other issues, as well as the infant's age and changes in feeding practices with age.

Several recent books explain life table and related multivariate analysis (Elandt-Johnson and Johnson, 1980; E. T. Lee, 1980), and computer programs are available. We will not examine in further detail the mechanics of such analyses. Some categorization schemes have tried to consider duration and degree of supplementation simultaneously, producing unordered, nonmutually exclusive categories and a loss of information; using life table and related multivariate analyses may eliminate such problems (e.g., Akin et al., 1981, 1985).

Where an infant-feeding practice is defined as a continuous variable (e.g., quantity of a particular item ingested, intensity of suckling, minutes spent feeding, days fed on a particular regimen) and such data can be collected, it is preferable to analyze the data using life table or regression analysis. If, in the analysis, logical thresholds or cutoff points appear, it may then be useful to categorize the data. Categorical analysis is simple, clear, and readily understood, as well as more suited to the data usually available. At present there is little theoretical basis for a particular categorization scheme, and categorical analysis does not allow the researcher to observe dose-response or threshold relationships. If categorical analysis is used, categories should preferably be ordered, equally incremented, mutually exclusive, and classified in a way which relates to the hypothesis being tested.

PROPOSED DEFINITIONS

The following definitions consider only the contrast between breast-feeding and all other infant-feeding practices; later in this section we discuss problems of categorizing other foods and practices. In both cases problems arise in formulating definitions applicable to a wide variety of research settings and goals. One problem has been the choice of a term to denote all infant-feeding practices other than breast-feeding, such as *breast milk substitutes*, *breast milk supplements*, *artificial feeding*, and *weaning foods*. Each term has connotations making it more suited to one particular set of hypotheses, and some terms suggest subsets rather than the whole group of infant-feeding practices other than breast-feeding. We use the term *other foods* throughout this book to encompass every infant diet other than breast-feeding that could introduce pathogens, affect infant appetite or growth, or alter time demands or hormonal effects on the mother. *Other foods* include any milk preparation, expressed breast milk, any juice or food, water, and vitamins. A term defined in such a general manner may result in problems, but it is convenient to our two sets of hypotheses.

When the term *other foods* seems clumsy or inappropriate, we may use *supplement*, *complement*, or *breast milk alternatives*. In all such cases the terms mean *all* other foods and not any particular subset. A particular example is the term *degree of supplementation*. This term, described below, refers to a continuum ranging from 0 to 100 percent supplementation, fully breast-fed to not breast-fed at all; in this sense, an infant's diet could be 100 percent supplements. Another example is the term *breast milk alternatives*, used to suggest the range of alternatives available to a mother in a given setting, but not to suggest that any particular feeding practice is an equivalent alternative to breast-feeding. At present no set of terms or definitions is entirely satisfactory; this is an area for further discussion.

Classification of Breast-Feeding Practices

These definitions emphasize the comparison of breast-feeding with other foods, although we are aware that other foods comprise a broad range of food sources that could be classified in many different ways. Later we will examine factors to consider in categorizing other foods; in this section, for convenience, we consider all other feeding patterns as one group of behaviors and practices that contrasts with breast-feeding.

Breast-feeding

Breast-feeding consists of the infant's suckling directly from the breast and ingesting the milk. The definition excludes the feeding of expressed breast milk because the process of expressing, bottling, and storing it may expose the infant to the same risk of contamination as a bottle-fed infant, and the interactional aspects of breast-feeding are completely lost, as are some of the immunological properties of breast milk (see chapter 4). Feeding expressed breast milk is fairly rare; it is usually to maintain the milk supply when breast-feeding cannot be accomplished (the infant is hospitalized or the mother works away from home). Exclusive breast-feeding means absolutely no other foods are used.

Partial or mixed breast-feeding

Sometimes called partial weaning, the category of partial or mixed breast-feeding encompasses the greatest range of behaviors and should be further subdivided into several categories. It would be desirable to consider the percentage of nutrients derived from breast-feeding, or the percentage of feedings that are breast-feedings. The difficulty of setting up a scale and measuring the degree of supplementation has resulted in one broad category which may include essentially full, partial, and minimal breast-feeders. Recording the number of breast-feedings and other feedings may give a crude measure of supplementation, which should be expressed as: (number of breast-feedings ÷ total number of feedings) × 100. The group may then be divided into percentiles (although there will be some artifactual heaping because total number of feedings are usually similar) from which a possible trend may be discovered. Preferably subdividing the mixed group should be based on objective, quantitative criteria—number of feedings, amount consumed, minutes spent at a feeding, type of supplement, or other point of prime interest to the researcher.

Duration of exclusive breast-feeding

Duration of exclusive breast-feeding refers to the number of days until the first other food (as defined above) is given.

Weaning

Roy E. Brown (1978) and John E. Gordon *et al*. (1963) suggest that when breast milk is taken as the normal food, any substitution for it is part of the weaning process. Infants never breast-fed are considered weaned at birth, and the weaning period is defined as the time during which breast milk is replaced by any other food.

Completely weaned

An infant is considered completely weaned after the first 24-hour period in which no breast-feeding takes place.

Nonbreast-fed

An infant is considered to be nonbreast-fed if it has not been breast-fed during the 24-hour period sampled.

Never breast-fed

The term *never breast-fed* refers to the infant who never received colostrum and has never been put to the breast.

Ever breast-fed

The term *ever breast-fed* is best used to describe the population of infants ever exposed to breast-feeding. In the broadest sense, it should include any infant ever put to the breast for whatever amount of time. Frequently, other operational definitions are used, defining an infant as ever breast-fed if, for example, it were being breast-fed on the day of discharge from the hospital. We prefer the first definition because it can be applied in any setting. The basic problem with the concept "ever breast-fed" is that it sets up a category embracing a very wide range of breast-feeding behaviors which may not be meaningful in some research settings. We suggest dealing with this problem by careful measurement of other breast-feeding characteristics (degree of supplementation or duration of breast-feeding).

The term *ever breast-fed* is often used to describe infants whose mothers "attempted" breast-feeding. Efforts to define groups of infants by their mother's decision to breast-feed or attempt at breast-feeding may be confusing. Are these two identical? How are these processes shown? What constitutes an attempt? Because of the subjective nature of these questions, we prefer using the term ever breast-fed, based on a measurable, distinct, observable behavior. We recommend that terms such as *attempted breast-feeding* or *decided to breast-feed* not be used to categorize mother-infant pairs.

The Immediate Postpartum Period

Studies of the first week of life particularly may need to record feeding practices on a day-by-day basis. Practices during this time vary considerably from one culture to another. Information regarding the following may be collected:

1. Other foods given before the first breast-feeding attempt.
2. Other foods given instead of colostrum.
3. Colostrum. Whether the infant receives colostrum or the mother expresses and discards it.
4. Coming-in of milk. Some medical texts describe the coming-in of breast milk as a discrete event (Vorherr, 1974); others indicate that the sudden and painful engorging of the breast with milk results from insufficient suckling in the immediate postpartum period (Newton and Newton, 1962). The breasts begin to produce milk instead of colostrum in the first few days postpartum, and the milk supply quickly increases, but it remains to be determined whether this change can be pinpointed to a specific day or hour, and whether it varies with culture, individual women, or practices of the first few days.
5. Other foods given before the coming-in of milk. In cultures where women feed other foods until the "milk comes in" and then breast-feed exclusively, the use of other foods before and after the milk comes in should be recorded as separate phenomena.

Classification of Other Foods

The group of other foods may be classified by any of the following criteria: liquids versus solids, milks versus nonmilks, home-prepared versus commercially prepared; economic cost to the family; protein, carbohydrate, lipid, mineral, and vitamin content; pathogen content.

Foods used as alternatives or supplements to breast milk vary greatly with cultural setting, season, and age of the infant. For example, Judith Johnston (1977) found 26 different infant diets observed during the first month of life among East Indians in Trinidad: combinations of breast milk, powdered milk, brown sugar, sago, Farax, diluted cow's milk, powdered milk with glucose, arrowroot, glucose, lime bud tea, green tea, flour pap, diluted evaporated milk, and diluted cow's milk with flour pap. In a large urban center in Honduras, over 80 percent of infants followed a complex pattern of using breast milk substitutes on a daily basis within two months of birth (O'Gara and Kendall, in press). Classifying other foods becomes more complex as the infant grows and gains access to more foods and in environments with a wide range of feeding choices. For these reasons most schemes classifying other foods will be specific to a particular study and hypothesis.

3
EFFECTS OF INFANT FEEDING ON INFANT HEALTH

This chapter introduces the effect of feeding on infant health. Figure III-1 depicts the relationship between groups of variables: independent, intervening, confounding, and outcome. Each block represents a category of variables which could be examined in further detail. Type of feeding refers to all possible infant-feeding practices and behaviors (chapter 2) considered as the independent variable throughout this book. Infant feeding may be conceptualized as affecting growth, morbidity, and mortality through three pathways. The intervening variables in these pathways are (1) exposure to pathogens, (2) infant's nutritional status, and (3) infant's immune status. These variables represent an intermediate level through which the causal agent (infant feeding) may affect growth, morbidity, and mortality. Figure III-1 also shows variables which may be considered confounders. Each group of variables is discussed further below.

INTERVENING VARIABLES

Exposure to Pathogens

Many factors affect the infant's level of exposure to pathogens. In our model, the term refers only to exposure as a consequence of feeding method and food preparation that is part of the feeding method. This model includes pathogens introduced by poor water supply or contamination of the feeding utensil and pathogen multiplication caused by inadequate food storage (e.g., lack of refrigeration). Where water quality and hygiene are good, and refrigeration is available, infant foods should not vary greatly in pathogen levels. In low-income settings, this pathway may assume greater importance in explaining differences in morbidity and mortality between breast-

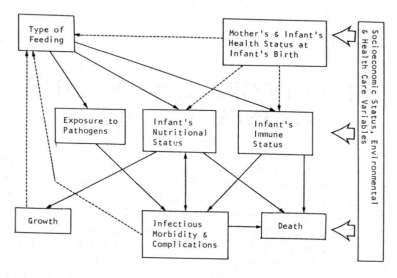

------ = confounding relationships

——— = pathways

FIGURE III-1   Factors affecting the relationship among infant feeding, growth, morbidity, and mortality.

fed and nonbreast-fed infants and among nonbreast-fed infants consuming various other foods.

Immune Status of the Infant

Immune status represents a hypothetical pathway by which infant feeding might affect morbidity and mortality. Infant-feeding practices may affect the infant's immunological capacity to respond to infection, most notably by providing active immunological components through breast-feeding. We discuss the contrast between breast-feeding and other infant-feeding practices and their impact on immune status in chapter 4. It seems plausible that the infant's immune status is an intervening variable when one compares morbidity and mortality in breast- and nonbreast-fed infants, but not an important variable when comparing nonbreast-fed infants to one another.

Breast milk is the only infant food which seems to affect infant immune status positively, by providing additional defenses against infection.

Nutritional Status

The term *nutritional status* has various connotations throughout the literature. We consider infant nutritional status to be the physical and biochemical characteristics resulting from feeding, independent of the effects of genetics or infectious disease. Nutritional status is considered good if it lets the infant grow and develop normally, although we are aware that "normal growth and development" have not been defined as well as might be desired. Nutritional status is a conceptual term, used to denote an intervening variable through which infant feeding may affect several outcomes, including growth, morbidity, and mortality.

OUTCOME VARIABLES

This book focuses on a series of outcomes—growth, infectious morbidity, and mortality—because of widespread concern about them, their public health importance, and the feasibility of measuring them.

Infectious Morbidity

This review is restricted to examining the relationship between infant feeding and infectious morbidity and excludes the relationship between infant feeding and noninfectious morbidity, such as allergic diseases (eczema, asthma, rhinitis, food allergy) or dental caries. We have also excluded outcomes of unclear etiology such as Sudden Infant Death Syndrome (SIDS), possible morbidity outcomes of later childhood or adulthood such as coronary artery disease, and psychological or developmental outcomes. In contrasting breast milk to other foods, the greatest evidence exists for the relationship between breast-feeding and infectious morbidity; evidence linking breast-feeding to other outcomes is much weaker. Further, infectious morbidity is of the greatest public health concern, particularly in low-income countries, and is thus the focus of our attention.

Death

The outcomes infectious morbidity and mortality are separated in figure III-1 because the pathways leading to morbidity may not be identical to those leading to mortality and the effect of infant feeding on each may be different. In our discussion of methodological issues, we point out the need for further clarification and specification of study outcomes, but in the epidemiological review we discuss morbidity and mortality studies in one group. Most published information has not distinguished between the various infectious outcomes or between the pathways leading to morbidity and mortality.

Growth

In keeping with our definition of nutritional status, growth is its main indicator. Biochemical indicators are also useful but because such measurements are generally expensive and invasive, they are less frequently used as indicators of nutritional status in epidemiological studies.

POTENTIAL CONFOUNDING VARIABLES

A *potential confounding variable* is one thought to be a determinant of the outcome of interest (morbidity, mortality, or growth) and to be unequally distributed among the exposed and the unexposed (e.g., different feeding methods) (Last, 1983). These associations may reflect underlying biological relationships or may be peculiarities of the data set; they may not necessarily pertain in all study populations. Some recent reviews and articles point out the need to control for confounding (Feachem and Koblinsky, 1984; Jason et al., 1984; Kovar et al., 1984), but there has been little mention of the need to assess confounding properly as part of the study design. Proper study design should provide plans to assess potential confounders, provide *a priori* criteria for designating them, and adequately control for existing confounding. Until now, overcontrol for confounding has not been a problem of studies examining the relationships among infant feeding, morbidity, mortality, and growth. Inappropriate or excessive controls for variables thought to be confounders can introduce biases, just as does insufficient control. Neither situation is desirable.

Below we describe several groups of variables that may be confounders in many environments. For possible relationships between these potential confounders and other study variables (exposure, intervening, and outcomes), see figure III-1. These hypothetical relationships remain to be examined in actual study settings.

A variable that confounds in one study or data set may not do so elsewhere. The following discussion highlights variables that would commonly be considered to be confounders in most studies, but in no way is a comprehensive list of all confounding variables. Further, the variables listed may not always be confounders.

Socioeconomic, Environmental, and Health Care Variables

The right side of figure III-1 indicates three broad categories of variables:

- Socioeconomic status and its correlates—occupation, income, educational level, neighborhood of residence; ethnic, racial, or cultural group
- Environmental variables—type of residence, number of people living in a room, water quality and supply, cooking and food storage facilities, general disease level in the population, climate, availability of food
- Health care variables—distance to nearest facility, economic cost, adequacy of care, availability of Western and non-Western types of care, practices and attitudes, cultural attitudes toward health and health care.

Each variable can be examined further. Most may affect each pathway in the model; many are intricately associated with each other. Many have been found to be associated with infant-feeding decisions, or strongly correlated with variables associated with type of infant-feeding method. Because these variables are so highly associated with each other, it may not be appropriate to control for all in any one study setting. The choice of which variables to assess or control for deserves careful thought and attention and must be specific to a study setting.

Health Status of Mother and Infant at Birth

Health status at birth refers to birth weight, gestational age, amount of maternal blood loss during delivery, level of anesthesia, maternal age, parity, and other factors thought to be associated with infant-feeding choices (particularly initiation of lactation) and with the infant's immune and nutritional status at birth and later.

Growth, Illness and Its Complications, and Their Interrelationships

The infant's condition at birth may affect feeding decisions, but it is equally likely that the infant's condition at any time after birth may affect such decisions. Illness or inappropriate growth as perceived by the mother, culture, or health care professional may lead to change in type or quantity of food given; these changes may vary with the culture and the illness. The effect of the infant's condition on feeding decisions has not been carefully measured or evaluated. It may be important to consider this relationship when attempting to show a causal effect of infant feeding on growth, morbidity, and mortality.

Clearly a variety of interrelated factors affect infant growth and the occurrence of infection. We are primarily concerned with examining the relationships among infant feeding, morbidity, mortality, and growth and suggest several pathways by which infant feeding may affect these outcomes. Extremely complex relationships have been simplified in order to examine these pathways. In chapter 4, we look at the pathways leading from infant feeding to immune status, morbidity, and death. We discuss immunological research regarding the effect of infant feeding on immune status, as well as factors which may affect immune status. We evaluate the epidemiological evidence to see whether an association between infant-feeding practices and morbidity and mortality is observed in populations of infants.

In chapter 5, we similarly examine the pathways leading from infant feeding to nutritional status and growth. We review the biochemical make-up of breast milk and other infant foods along with their potential effects on nutritional status and epidemiological studies examining the relationship between infant feeding and growth.

The interrelationships among nutritional status, immune status, morbidity, and growth are discussed briefly in chapter 6. In chapters 4 and 5 we consider nutritional status to be a confounding variable when morbidity and mortality are the outcome variables, and morbidity to be a confounding variable when growth is the outcome variable. This convenient separation belies the complexity of the situation. Eventually researchers will have to consider more carefully the interrelationships among these variables and the intricate pathways involved.

We give insufficient attention to the pathway leading from infant feeding to exposure to pathogens, thus to morbidity and mortality, and we do not attempt to hypothesize the relative importance of any pathway. We suggest that infant feeding may affect morbidity and mortality by affecting the infant's immune status, level of exposure to pathogens, or nutritional status, which in turn may affect immune status. We also suggest that infant feeding may affect growth through affecting nutritional status or by affecting levels of morbidity, which in turn influence nutritional status and growth. We review biological evidence regarding the plausibility of such pathways, and epidemiological evidence of associations among infant feeding and growth, morbidity, and mortality. Future researchers may want to evaluate the relative importance of each pathway or elucidate other pathways.

4
INFANT FEEDING AND MORBIDITY

IMMUNOLOGICAL EVIDENCE

The hypothesized immunologic protection of human milk is an important factor consistently referred to in support of breast-feeding (Butler, 1979; France *et al.*, 1980; Hanson and Winberg, 1972). Issues in evaluating these benefits include:

1. *Capacity of fetus, neonate, and infant to protect themselves immunologically.* This basic information allows independent assessment of the effects of type of feeding on the infant's ability to protect itself and also helps determine how essential human milk is for infants.

2. *Factors that may affect capacity of neonate and infant to protect themselves immunologically.* To differentiate among the effects of type of feeding and other variables (confounding relationships) on the functional capacity of the infant's immune system, it may be necessary to adjust for them in research design and data analysis.

3. *Possible mechanisms by which protective constituents in human milk alter infant's susceptibility to infection.* Understanding these mechanisms may provide a biologically plausible link between type of feeding and effects on infant health and may also allow speculation about which biologic system may be affected most in terms of morbidity and its complications.

Development of the Immune System

Definitions of elements of immunity

The immunological system is the principal means of defense against foreign agents such as pathogenic organisms and macromolecules like large fibrous

27

and globular proteins. An immune response consists of the formation of specific proteins (antibodies) and the activation of cells to react with and eliminate foreign agents which might otherwise harm the host. Foreign agents eliciting an immune response are collectively known as antigens (Ags). The immune response is mediated through two separate, but related pathways—the humoral and cell-mediated responses.

Humoral responses involve the action of specific serum proteins against antigens. These proteins, known as antibodies (Abs), belong to a special group of serum proteins called immunoglobulins (IgA, IgD, IgE, IgG, and IgM).

Cell-mediated responses are reactions of certain classes of cells (lymphocytes and macrophages) to the presence of antigen. Two main types of lymphocytes are involved in the immune response: B lymphocytes arising from a stem cell in the fetal liver and in the bone marrow of adults, and T lymphocytes which mature in the thymus gland. When triggered by an antigen, B lymphocytes divide and the daughter cells synthesize and secrete antibody molecules. T lymphocytes react in several ways to antigen presence. Some are "killer cells" that destroy target cells (e.g., bacteria) with appropriate surface antigens. Other T lymphocytes produce substances causing local inflammation (delayed-type hypersensitivity), which halts the spread of infectious agents. Still others control the responses of other antigen-triggered lymphocytes, either as helpers that promote the maturation of antigen-stimulated B and T cells or as suppressors that block the enhancing activity of the T helpers.

Other accessory components of the immune system include the polymorphonuclear leukocytes, neutrophils, and macrophage. In a very general sense, epithelial and endodermal cells may also be considered part of the immune system because of their role in protecting the organism from the external environment (Butler, 1979).

A detailed description of these elements is readily available in many textbooks (Bellanti, 1985; Benacerraf and Unanue, 1979). In several tables we summarize the presence and capacity of the elements providing immunity at different ages.

Fetal immune status

Prenatally, the fetus predominantly receives IgG antibodies. Mothers with high amounts (titers) of circulating antibodies provide good protection against infection to their infants (table IV-1), while mothers with low titers protect their babies only partially or very poorly. Passively transferred anti-

TABLE IV-1

Neonatal passive immunity: placental passage of maternal antibodies

Passive Transfer		
Good (IgG)	Poor	None (mostly IgM)
Antinulcear Ab (ANA)	*Beta pertussis* Ab	*Escherichia coli* H and O Ab
Antistaphylolysin Ab	*Hemophilus influenzae* Ab	Heterophile Ab
Antistreptolysin Ab	*Shigella flexneri* Ab	Natural (anti-A, anti-B)
Beta pertussis agglutinin	*Streptococcus* MG Ab	isoagglutinins
Diphtheria antitoxin		Reaginic Ab (IgE)
Group B streptococcal Ab		Rh saline (complete)
Immune (anti-A, anti-B)		isoagglutinins
isoagglutinins		*Salmonella somatic* (O) Ab
Long-acting thyroid stimulator		Wasserman Ab
Measles Ab		
Mumps Ab		
Poliomyelitis Ab		
Rh incomplete (Coombs') Ab		
Salmonella flagellar (H) Ab		
Tetanus antitoxin		
VDRL Ab		

Source: Adapted from Michael Miller and Richard Stiehm, "Immunology and Resistance to Infection," in *Infectious Diseases of the Fetus and Newborn Infant*, edited by Jack S. Remington and Jerome O. Klein, 2d ed., Saunders, Philadelphia, 1983, table 1, with permission.

bodies decline progressively postnatally depending on three factors: (1) initial concentration, (2) degradative activity, and (3) antibody half-life. Detailed analyses of diptheria toxin indicate that the decline follows an exponential function with a half-life of about four weeks (Dixon *et al.*, 1952). Lack of transmission of IgM across the placenta may explain neonates' susceptibility to infection by gram-negative organisms such as *E. coli* and *Salmonella* (Gitlin *et al.*, 1963). IgG antibodies directed against their somatic antigen (Cohen and Norins, 1968) may provide partial protection against these organisms, indicating the capability of fetal B cells to produce antibody when stimulated. See table IV-2.

Placental structure partially determines prenatal transfer of immunity. In humans, as pregnancy advances the thickness of the placental layers decreases with an increase in capillarization which may cause the increase in immunoglobulin transfer seen as pregnancy progresses. Premature infants

TABLE IV-2

Presence and capacity of immune system during gestation and neonatal period

Type of Immunity	Fetus		Neonate (0–28 days old)	
	Presence	Capacity	Presence	Capacity
Cellular Elements				
B lymphocytes				
Stem cell	Detected at 8 wks[1]	Capable of differentiating without B cells	Present	
Immature	Detected at 9 wks[1]	Susceptible to inactivation or induction of tolerance[1]	Present	Diminished immunoglobulin production: see humoral elements
Mature	Detected at 10–12 wks; bear IgA, IgG, IgM[1]	Limited Ab production on stimulation; predominantly IgM[6]	Normal; increased %age of EAC-binding lymphocytes[8]	
T lymphocytes	Detected at 8–9 wks in thymus;[2] develop specific antigenic markers[3]	Induce graft-vs-host reaction;[7] possible antiviral T-mediated mechanism	Decreased %age of E-binding lymphocytes[8]	Suppress B cell differentiation & Ab synthesis;[14] decreased cytotoxic & lytic activity;[15] strong proliferative response to mitogens;[23] lymphotoxin production about 40% of adult level[23]

TABLE IV-2 (continued)

Type of Immunity	Fetus		Neonate (0–28 days old)	
	Presence	Capacity	Presence	Capacity
Phagocytic system	Little known	Little known	Possibly immature macrophage	Depressed monocyte-marcrophage system;[16] diminished phagocytosis;[17] diminished bacteri-cidal or viricidal activity;[18] less effective PMN migrating capacity,[19] normal PMN phagocytic & bactericidal activity[20]
Humoral Elements Immunoglobulins				
IgA	No placental transfer	—	$1 \pm 2\%$ of adult level[9]	First detected in intestine at wk 4[23]
IgD	No placental transfer	—	1% of adult level[10]	—
IgE	No placental transfer	—	1% of adult level[11]	Appears around wk 4[23]
IgG	Placentally transferred;[4] minimal endogenous synthesis	Passive immunity	$89 \pm 17\%$ of adult level,[9] passively acquired	Protects against specific Ag; inhibits active AB production[21]

TABLE IV-2 (continued)

Type of Immunity	Fetus		Neonate (0–28 days old)	
	Presence	Capacity	Presence	Capacity
IgM	Detected at 30 wks; no placental transfer	Protection during congenital infection	$11 \pm 5\%$ of adult level;[9] endogenous production	—
Complement	No placental transfer;[5] synthesized early	—	C3, C4, C5: 55–60% of adult levels[12]	Deficient opsonic activity[22]
Organ Thymus	Originates at 6 wks[2]	Develops lymphoid cells at 8–9 wks[2]	About 33% of adult size $(10–15 \text{ g})$[13]	—

Sources: (1) Lawton & Cooper, 1979; (2) Stites & Pavia, 1979; (3) Janossy et al., 1980; (4) Gitlin et al., 1964; (5) Gitlin & Biasucci, 1969; (6) Fudenberg et al., 1980; (7) Asantila et al., 1973; (8) Fleischer et al., 1975; (9) Steihm & Fudenberg, 1966; (10) Josephs & Buckley, 1980; (11) Bazaral et al., 1971; (12) Miller, 1978; (13) Bellanti and Kadlec, 1985; (14) Abedin & Kirkpatrick, 1980; (15) Lubens et al., 1980; (16) Poplack & Blaese, 1980; (17) Bellanti et al., 1979; (18) Sullivan et al., 1975; (19) Miller, 1971; (20) Park et al., 1970; (21) Evans & Smith, 1963; (22) Dossett et al., 1969; (23) Miller & Stiehm, 1983.

Notes: — = data unavailable or inconclusive

may therefore be at a disadvantage so far as this function is concerned (Vahlquist, 1958).

T cells are probably only partially functional in the human fetus, although evidence of functioning T cells exists in animal fetuses. Fetal lambs have been known to reject skin grafts during gestation (Silverstein and Prendergast, 1964). Little is known about development of the monocyte-phagocyte system. (See table IV-2 for the functional capacity of T cells and the phagocytic system in the neonate.)

An important finding of Lubens and coworkers (1980) requiring further investigation is the decreased cytotolic activity of T lymphocytes in infants and children under age two. Percentage lysis of [51]chromium-labelled EL4 cells was used as an index of the level of cytotoxicity of T lymphocytes at various ages. The decreased chemotactic ability of polymorphonuclear and mononuclear leukocytes may in turn depress delayed hypersensitivity skin tests and inflammatory reactions, thereby increasing neonatal and infantile susceptibility to infection (Klein, et al., 1977). In addition, deficient bactericidal capacity for *E. coli* in the newborn (Dossett et al., 1969) may contribute to increased susceptibility to infection, especially by gram-negative organisms.

Development of the human immune system differs from that of other animals, especially in the amount of antibodies transferred across the placenta to the fetus, which subsequently determines the significance of antibody ingested via colostrum and milk (table IV-3). For example, hoofed animals have no significant placental transfer of antibody, so the immunity then obtained via colostrum and milk is essential. Absence of this immunity is life threatening. Because significant amounts of immune elements are transferred to the human fetus prenatally, the importance and essentiality of colostrum and breast milk in rendering immunity can be questioned. The value of immunity through colostrum is obviously different for human babies and the young hoofed animal; but comparing the infant's immune status with that of an adult, the infant appears fairly naive and may indeed benefit from the protective factors found in breast milk. See table IV-4 and figure IV-1.

Neonatal immune status (0–28 days postpartum)

Throughout gestation normal development continues in a protected environment. This factor coupled with the incomplete development of immune tissue (e.g., thymus), the presence of placentally transferred immunosuppressive antibodies, and B cell hyporesponsiveness make the newborn

TABLE IV-3

Acquisition of immunity

Animal	No. of Placental Layers	Importance of Antibody Transfer	
		Placental	Colostrum
Man	3	+	–
Rat & mouse	4	+	–
Dog & cat	5	+	–
Cow	5	–	+
Horse	6	–	+

Source: Adapted from Bellanti (1985), p. 48.
Notes: + = transfer of antibodies essential for survival;
— = importance of transfer questionable—negligible in case of cow and horse

TABLE IV-4

Presence and capacity of immune system in the adult

Type of Immunity	Presence	Capacity
Cellular Elements		
B lymphocytes	5% of total lymphocytes; surface molecules include: immunoglobulin C3 receptors; Fc receptors; histocompatibility molecules	Mature into plasma cells which produce immunoglobulins Transplantation immunity
T lymphocytes	80–90% of total lymphocytes; histocompatibility molecules; T cell-specific molecules	Modulate activity of B cells & other T cells; delayed type hypersensitivity; contact sensitivity; transplantation immunity; cytotoxic T cells (capacity to kill other cells)
Phagocytic system	Main component: macrophage which constitutes scavenger reticuloendothelial system	Endocytosis; pinocytosis; phagocytosis; intracellular digestion; interaction with B & T cells in immune response
Humoral Elements		
Immunoglobulins		
IgA	250 mg/dl	TN, A, opsonization (?)
IgD	3 mg/dl	Antigen receptor on B cell
IgE	.01 mg/dl	Mediates changes in vascular permeability
IgG	1100 mg/dl	TN, A, B, . . .; opsonization
IgM	100 mg/dl	Toxin neutralization; agglutination; bacterolytic with complement; antigen receptor on B cell
Complement	Series of 14 proteins	React with Ab-Ag complexes, exert their effect primarily on cell membranes, causing lysis or cellular aberration
Organ		
Thymus	Reaches maximum size at age 4–5 (30–40 g)	Generates T cells

Source: Benacerraf & Unanue, 1979.
Notes: A = agglutination; B = bacterolytic with complement; TN = toxin neutralization

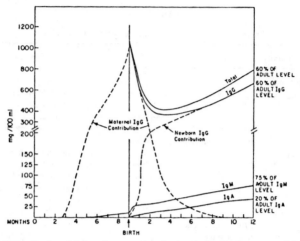

FIGURE IV-1   Fetal and infant immunoglobulin levels in the first year of life. Source: Adapted from Michael Miller and Richard Stiehm, "Immunology and Resistance to Infection," in *Infectious Diseases of the Fetus and Newborn Infant*, edited by Jack S. Remington and Jerome O. Klein, 2d ed., Saunders, Philadelphia, 1983, figure 5, with permission. Copyright W. B. Saunders Co.

relatively defenseless against the extrauterine environment. After birth the infant immune system continues to develop but several constituents do not reach adult levels until well past infancy (e.g., thymus). See table IV-5.

Since IgG is acquired transplacentally, it predominates during the period immediately after birth. IgM rises rapidly during the fourth and seventh days of life, while IgA is present only in very small amounts. Bacterial colonization of the gastrointestinal tract soon after birth is an important factor in stimulating production of immunoglobulins.

The effect of prenatally acquired immunoglobulin is also observed during the neonatal period. This phenomenon has been studied in neonates and infants who have been immunized and those who possess high levels of passively acquired antibodies.

Infantile immune status

An infant can produce antibodies, although the level is not yet clearly defined. The relation between the infant's age and ability to produce antibody has been most often studied in clinical immunization trials. Osborn

TABLE IV-5

Presence and capacity of immune system during infancy

Type of Immunity	Age 28 days–6 months		Age 6–12 months	
	Presence	Capacity	Presence	Capacity
Cellular Elements				
B lymphocytes	Present	Synthesis of Ig classes	Present	Synthesis of Ig classes
T lymphocytes	Present	Decreased delayed cutaneous hypersensitivity & cytotoxicity	Present	Decreased cytotoxicity
Phagocytic system	—	Decreased PMN & mononuclear chemotaxis[1]	—	Same[1]
Humoral Elements				
Immunoglobulins				
IgA	14 ± 9% of adult levels[2]	—	19 ± 9% of adult levels[2]	—
IgD	Present	—	Present	—
IgE	Present	—	30% of adult level[3]	—
IgG	37 ± 10% of adult levels	—	58 ± 19% of adult levels	—
IgM	43 ± 17% of adult levels	—	55 ± 23% of adult levels	—
Complement	Present	—	Present	—
Organ				
Thymus	At 6 wks gestation	—	Present	—

Sources: (1) Klein *et al.*, 1977; (2) Stiehm & Fudenberg, 1966; (3) Bazaral *et al.*, 1971; (4) Miller & Stiehm, 1983.
Notes: — = data unavailable or inconclusive for this age group; PMN = polymorphonuclear leukocytes

and colleagues (1952) studied the response of infants (who had no circulating antitoxin) to a single injection of high-titer diphtheria or tetanus toxoid (see figures IV-2 and IV-3). Young infants did not respond as quickly with antibody production and did not reach the antitoxin level of older infants. The study of Osborn *et al.* suggests that the infant's response to diphtheria and tetanus toxoid improves with age, although the amount of antitoxin

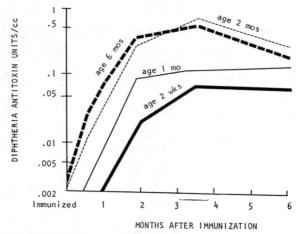

FIGURE IV-2   Diphtheria immunization: Mean response of infants of different age groups with antitoxin titer graphed on logarithmic scale. Source: Adapted from John J. Osborn, Joseph Dancis, and Juan F. Julia, "Studies of the Immunology of the Newborn Infant. 1. Age and Antibody Production," *Pediatrics* 9, no. 6, June 1952, p. 738, with permission. Copyright American Academy of Pediatrics.

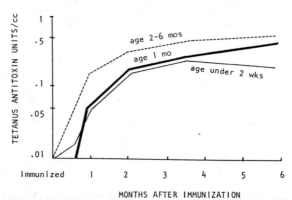

FIGURE IV-3   Tetanus immunization: Mean response of infants of different age groups with antitoxin titer graphed on logarithmic scale. Source: Adapted form John J. Osborn, Joseph Dancis, and Juan F. Julia, "Studies of the Immunology of the Newborn Infant. 1. Age and Antibody Production," *Pediatrics* 9, no. 6, June 1952, p. 741, with permission. Copyright American Academy of Pediatrics.

produced at all ages was considered protective. These data reaffirm that infants are capable of forming antibody to tetanus and diphtheria toxoid at birth, and this ability improves throughout infancy. Although we have no *direct* evidence that maternal antibody suppresses the neonate's responses to antigen, this phenomenon has been implicated in the decreased response of neonates to immunization against infectious diseases. How maternal antibody acts in a suppressive manner is unclear (Evans and Smith, 1963).

Another phenomenon observed in infancy is physiologic hypogamma-globulinemia—normally low immunoglobulin levels (Kaur *et al.*, 1979; Miller and Stiehm, 1983). Immunoglobulin levels are at their lowest at about four to six months of age. At this time, prenatally transferred anti-bodies have presumably decreased to insignificant levels and the infant, if not exposed to antigens, has low levels of actively produced Igs—so the young infant *may* be more susceptible to infection. The suppressive activity found in the newborn, if prolonged, may also contribute to hypogamma-globulinemia.

Factors affecting immune status

Figure IV-4 presents factors affecting immune status, focusing on the re-lationship between health/nutritional status and immune status.

There is considerable evidence that nutrient deficiencies interfere with the immune response, both humoral and cell-mediated (R. L. Gross and Newberne, 1980). Maternal malnutrition during gestation and altered nu-tritional status of the infant may affect immunocompetence. Kaur *et al.* (1979) assessed the immune status of preterm and small-for-date (SFD) babies at birth, three, and six months of age in comparison to full-term (weight appropriate for gestational age) controls (table IV-6). The lower IgG levels observed in SFD and preterm newborns may be attributed to deprivation of transplacentally transferred IgG, which usually increases during the last trimester of preganacy. The increased IgG levels at six months may have resulted from subclinical infections.

Other studies (Bhaskaram *et al.*, 1977; Jagadeesan and Reddy, 1978; Ueda *et al.*, 1980a,b) indicate similar results, and generally conclude that birth weight, gestational age, and maternal nutritional status (which influ-ences birth weight) are related to infant immune status. Of the above factors, most certain is the relationship between nutritional and immune status. The other linkages require further research.

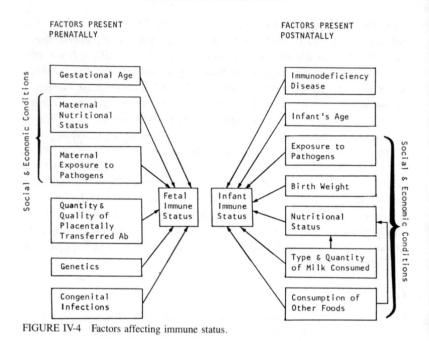

FIGURE IV-4   Factors affecting immune status.

TABLE IV-6

Immunologic response of small-for-date (SFD) and preterm (PT)
babies compared to controls

Immunologic Response	Birth		3 months		6 months	
	SFD	PT	SFD	PT	SFD	PT
Complement (C3)	↓	↓	C	C	C	C
Cell-mediated immunity	↓	↓	↓	C	↓	C
IgA	↓	↓	↓	C	C	C
IgG	↓	↓	C	C	↑	↑
IgM	↓	↓	↓	C	C	C

Source: Kaur *et al.*, 1979.
Notes: C = levels comparable to controls; ↓ = level lower than controls; ↑ = level higher than controls

Summary and conclusions

Although complete information is not yet available on all components of the immune system, it is recognized that the immune system is not fully developed at birth and continues to be immature throughout infancy. Of particular concern are the low levels of IgA, IgE, and IgM at birth and the decline in circulating levels of IgG after birth before the infant's own production fully compensates for the decline in maternally contributed IgG. As figure IV-1 indicates, total immunoglobulin levels are lowest from two to six months of age. Of course, it is not known whether these low levels are due to an immature immune system or to lack of exposure to antigens.

Antimicrobial Factors in Human Milk

Human milk contains a spectrum of interacting specific and nonspecific resistance factors believed to provide the immune protection associated with breast-feeding. We review them as a first step in showing how infant-feeding patterns may affect infant health status.

Antimicrobial resistance factors in milk include: (1) cellular components such as T and B lymphocytes, macrophages, and neutrophils; (2) the immunoglobulins, IgA, IgD, IgE, IgG, and IgM; and (3) elements other than immunoglobulins or cells, such as complement, interferon, iron-binding proteins, lysozyme, bifidus factor, and antistaphylococcal factor.

There is a great deal of individual variation in amounts of these protective factors present and in the biochemical quality of human colostrum and milk. These differences may be attributed to the mother's nutritional and health status (Miranda et al., 1983), emotional status, state of hydration, and presence or absence of infection (Pittard, 1979). Differences in techniques used to detect the amounts of these constituents, and timing of these measurements, may also influence differences observed.

Cellular components

Quantification of the cellular elements in colostrum and milk requires further investigation. It is presently thought that the predominant cells are T and B lymphocytes and macrophages (table IV-7). Function(s) of these cells have been studied in vitro (table IV-8), and since they are probably not absorbed in the gut, one may speculate that they function on the local environment.

TABLE IV-7

Concentration and survival of antimicrobial components in human milk

Component	Concentration		Adult Serum (9)	GI Tract Survival	Percentage Loss in Storage		
	Colostrum	Milk			Pasteurization @63°C	Lyophilization (4)	Freezing (4)
Cellular Elements							
B lymphocytes	34% of lymphocytes (1)	—	5% of lymphocytes	?	100 (4)	100	100
T lymphocytes	50% of lymphocytes (1) 10^5/ml (2)	$10^4 - 10^2$/ml (2)	80–90% of lymphocytes	?	100 (4)	100	100
Macrophages	2.1×10^6/ml	$6-1.3 \times 10^5$/ml	—	?	—	—	—
Neutrophils	—	2.1×10^6/ml	—	?	—	—	—
Immunoglobulins							
IgA	126 mg/dl (4) 600 mg/dl (5)	36.5 mg/dl (4) 80 mg/dl (5)	250 mg/dl	+(10)	33 (4)	21	0
IgD	—	—	3 mg/dl	—	—	—	—
IgE	—	—	.01 mg/dl	—	—	—	—
IgG	6.7 mg/dl (4) 80 mg/dl (5)	1.8 mg/dl (4) 16 mg/dl (5)	1100 mg/dl	—	50 (4)	75	50

TABLE IV-7 (continued)

| Component | Concentration | | | GI Tract Survival | Percentage loss in Storage | | |
	Colostrum	Milk	Adult Serum (9)		Pasteurization @63°C	Lyophilization (4)	Freezing (4)
IgM	14.7 mg/dl (4) 125 mg/dl (5)	2.1 mg/dl (4) 30 mg/dl (5)	10 mg/dl	Labile	40 (4)	90	100
Complement	4.4 mg/dl (6)	0–2.8 mg/dl (6)	—	?	—	—	—
Interferon	—	—	—	—	—	—	—
Lactoferrin	420 mg/dl (7)	250 mg/dl (7) 370 mg/dl (8)	—	+	70 (8)	—	—
Lysozyme	14.2 mg/dl (7)	24.8 mg/dl (7) 39 mg/dl (8)	—	+(11)	0 (8)	—	—
Bifidus factor	—	—	—	—	—	—	—
Antistaphylo-coccal factor	—	—	—	—	—	—	—

Sources: (1) Diaz-Jouanen & Williams, 1974; (2) Ogra & Ogra, 1978; (3) Pitt, 1979; (4) Liebhaber, 1977; (5) Michael *et al.*, 1971; (6) Mata & Wyatt, 1971; (7) Reddy *et al.*, 1977; (8) Ford *et al.*, 1977; (9) Fudenberg *et al.*, 1980; (10) Tomasi & Beinenstock, 1968; (11) Jollès & Jollès, 1961.

Notes: — = data unavailable or inconclusive; + = component survives in gastrointestinal tract

TABLE IV-8

Mechanisms of action of antimicrobial components in human milk

Component	Proposed Function
Cellular Elements	
B lymphocytes	Synthesize immunoglobulin[1]
T lymphocytes	Diminished response to phytohemaglutinin[2] ⟶ decreased production of immunologic mediator(s); produces: (a) lymphocyte-derived chemotactic factor to attract monocytes to mucosal surface; (b) interferon as defense against virus
Macrophage	Synthesizes lysozyme;[3] produces complement proteins (C4);[2] increases giant cell formation[4] ⟶ increased phagocytic activity; interacts with lymphocytes;[5] release of intracellular IgA into tissue culture[6] ⟶ transport vehicle for immunoglobulin release
Polymorphonuclear leukocytes	Increased metabolic & phagocytic activity[7]
Immunoglobulin IgA	Binds pathogenic bacteria;[8] coats bacteria;[9] binds to secretory component on mucosal surface in gut & oral cavities;[10] protects against dietary antigens;[11] rotavirus and other bacterial neutralizing activity
Complement	Promotes opsonization: activated by the alternate pathway, initiated by IgA (Ia) or classical pathway[12]
Interferon	—
Lactoferrin	Iron chelator ⟶ inhibits bacterial growth
Lysozyme	Lyses bacterial cell wall
Bifidus factor	Enhances lactobacillus bifidus colonization ⟶ lowered pH in gut ⟶ inhibits colonization of intestine by enteric pathogens
Antistaphylococcal factor	Inhibits staphylococcal infection

Sources: (1) Murillo & Goldman, 1970; (2) Ogra & Ogra, 1978; (3) Pitt, 1979; (4) Smith & Goldman, 1971; (5) Nelson & Leu, 1975; (6) Pittard et al., 1977; (7) Johnson et al., 1980; (8) McClelland et al., 1972; (9) Williams & Gibbons, 1972; (10) Roberts et al., 1980; (11) Hanson et al., 1977; (12) Boackel et al., 1974.

Note: — = data unavailable or inconclusive

T lymphocytes from milk act differently from blood T cells from the same donor (Parmely et al., 1976). For example, milk T cells were unresponsive to *Candida albicans* although blood T cells were not; milk T cells responded to the K capsular antigen for *E. coli*, while blood lymphocytes showed minimal response. This response difference may indicate capability of lacteal tissue to select populations of immunocompetent cells. Thus, milk lymphocytes express a select set of responses not always representative of peripheral immunity in the host. Studies by Mohr *et al.* (1970) and Ogra *et al.* (1977) indicate that T lymphocytes may also be involved in the transfer of cell-mediated immunity, and delayed hypersensitivity via subcellular components of immune lymphocytes (Diaz-Jouanen and Williams, 1974). Further investigation is necessary to determine how milk lymphocytes influence the development and functional capacity of the neonate and infant immune system.

In addition to the functions mentioned in table IV-8, Pittard *et al.* (1977) suggest that macrophages may be involved in the transport of immunoglobulins, especially IgA.

B cells in milk are similar to T cells in probably representing a subpopulation of cells different from peripheral blood. Milk B lymphocytes lack complement receptors, represent a larger proportion of the total lymphocyte count, and are enriched with surface IgA compared to blood lymphocytes.

Immunoglobulins

Secretory IgA (sIgA) is the predominant immunoglobulin in milk (table IV-7). The concentration of all the immunoglobulins decreases from colostrum to milk although there is an increase in milk volume with prolonged lactation which compensates for the decrease. The predominance of IgA in human milk (as opposed to other immunoglobulins) has not yet been clearly explained. IgG is transplacentally transferred, and in conjunction with IgM is the predominant immunoglobulin found in infant sera. IgA is not transferred through the placenta and is present at low levels in infant sera, but is the predominant immunoglobulin in human milk. Does it provide a level of protection otherwise normally lacking? How does an infant not consuming human milk compensate for this deficiency? These questions can only be answered through further research. The function of the secretory component of IgA remains to be determined. It has been proposed that it may increase resistance of IgA to proteolysis or aid in transport of IgA (as cited in Larson and Smith by Butler, 1979). Immunoelectron microscopy has been used to study localization of IgA and IgM in human colostrum. Moro *et al.* (1983) present data indicating that these immunoglobulins are not synthesized by lymphoid cells in colostrum but are acquired by phagocytic cells and noncellular globules. The origin of sIgA and its mechanism of release has been further studied (Halsey *et al.*, 1983; Weaver *et al.*, 1984), but is beyond the realm of this book.

Unlike the case of the rat and piglet, human colostral and milk immunoglobulins are thought not to be absorbed from the intestine (Ammann and

Stiehm, 1966; Yap *et al.*, 1979) although S. S. Ogra *et al.* (1977) and Roberts and Freed (1977) present contrary evidence. Table IV-8 provides information on the proposed function and mechanism of action of human milk immunoglobulins.

The majority of pathogens for which human milk contains antibodies are specific for enterobacterial agents (see table IV-9). This specificity is currently attributed to the "homing" phenomenon, in which maternal B cells in intestinal Peyer's patches, after being "sensitized" by gut antigens, migrate to the mucosal surface lining exocrine glands, such as the breast (Head and Beer, 1978). Consequently, colostrum and milk contain antibodies directed against maternal intestinal flora that are likely to be similar to organisms in the infant's system, and thereby provide local protection against these microbes. Glass *et al.* (1983) offer evidence for the presence of IgA antibodies against cholera toxin and lipopolysaccharides. The interesting aspect of this protection is its apparent inability to protect children against colonization with *Vibrio cholerae* although it did protect those colonized with the organism against diarrheal disease. Also, although some studies have indicated that human milk provides protection against rotavirus (table IV-9), more recent studies disagree with these findings (Berger *et al.*, 1983; Totterdell *et al.*, 1980, 1982). We discuss the benefits and hazards of ingested immunoglobulin below.

TABLE IV-9

Organisms against which protection has been demonstrated in human milk

Organism	Study
Brucellus abortus	Coombs *et al.*, 1983
Corynebacterium diphtheriae	Goldman & Smith, 1973
Coxsackie virus (B3, B5, A9); Echo virus (6, 9)	Michaels, 1965
Escherichia coli	Coombs *et al.*, 1983; Dolby & Stephens, 1983; Kenny *et al.*, 1967
Group B streptococci	Coombs *et al.*, 1983
Hemophilus pertussis	Adams *et al.*, 1947
Pneumococcus	Mouton *et al.*, 1970
Polio virus (1, 2, 3)	Warren *et al.*, 1964
Rotavirus	Inglis *et al.*, 1978; Otnaess & Orstavik, 1980; Simhon *et al.*, 1979; Totterdell *et al.*, 1983
Staphylococcus aureus	Nordbring, 1957
Streptococcus mutans	Arnold *et al.*, 1976; Eggert & Gurner, 1984

An important factor that may influence the level of immunoglobulins in milk is maternal malnutrition, although data on this subject are controversial. Reddy and colleagues (1977) found no significant differences in the levels of milk immunoglobulins, lysozyme, lactoferrin, hemoglobin, and serum albumin among well-nourished and undernourished Indian women, but McMurray *et al.* (1981) noted signficantly lower colostrum levels of IgA and IgG, albumin, and C4 (complement protein) among undernourished Colombian women. Suzuki and colleagues (1983) and Lewis-Jones and Reynolds (1983) report higher levels of IgA and other antimicrobial proteins in early preterm human milk compared to term human milk, possibly an important advantage to preterm infants allowed to breast-feed. Although levels of these proteins are higher in preterm milk, Murphy *et al.* (1983) present evidence to show that the antimicrobial properties of preterm breast milk cells are the same as term milk. Their ability to phagocytize and kill staphylococci was the same. In addition, Prentice *et al.* (1983a) consider parity the major determinant of the level of protective factors produced in milk of rural Gambian women.

Elements other than immunoglobulins and cells

Complement

A series of 14 proteins constitute and are involved in the complement pathway. Their effect is primarily on cell membranes, causing lysis of some cells and functional aberrations in others. They also mediate other activities such as opsonization, chemotaxis, and the release of allergic effectors, as well as activating B lymphocytes and macrophages. Complement protein C3 is an essential component involved in both activation pathways.

The susceptibility of complement to inactivation by gastric contents allows question of its role in establishing gastrointestinal immunity. The two possible modes of action of complement in milk are questionable (table IV-8). Boackel *et al.* (1974) suggest that sIgA interacts with complement thereby exerting its opsonizing/lytic activity at mucosal surfaces (e.g., gastrointestinal and respiratory tracts).

Iron-binding proteins

Human milk contains large amounts of the iron-chelating protein lactoferrin (table IV-7), is less than 50 percent saturated with iron, and acts by making iron unavailable to bacteria for multiplication (table IV-8) (J. J. Bullen *et al.*, 1972). Recent evidence indicates that lactoferrin may bind to the secretory component of IgA and be released by cleavage of disulfide bonds. Since both IgA and lactoferrin are known to participate in the bacteriostatic activity of human milk, and lactoferrin also enhances this antibacterial activity in the presence of IgA (Bullen *et al.*, 1972), it would be interesting and worthwhile to investigate further the significance of the binding of lactoferrin to IgA. In addition, both lactoferrin and IgA levels ingested per day decline over the first four months of life and are closely correlated with the infant's increased production of sIgA (Butte *et al.*, 1984b).

Lysozyme

This enzyme is capable of lysing bacteria (table IV-8) and is stable in the acidic gastric environment. Its concentration in milk increases with prolonged lactation (table IV-7) (Butte *et al.*, 1984b).

Bifidus factor

The quality of colonization by intestinal flora in breast-fed infants is distinctively different from that of infants fed cow's milk or infant formula. Breast-fed infants are rapidly colonized with *Lactobacillus bifidus* while infants fed cow's milk develop a mixed intestinal flora (Beerens *et al.* 1980). Colonization by *L. bifidus* is considered beneficial to the infant's health (see below). The ability of breast-fed infants to encourage the growth of *L. bifidus* is partially attributable to the bifidus factor. See table IV-8 for its mode of action, particularly suppression of gut colonization by gram-negative organisms such as *E. coli*.

Other factors

Besides the protective factors mentioned above, Holmgren and colleagues (1983) present data on receptor-like glycocompounds in human milk with the ability to prevent bacterial (*El Tor Vibrio cholerae*) adherence by competition with receptors on target cells. This organism is an important cause of diarrhea and colonizes the intestinal epithelium. Inhibiting adherence of the bacteria to its target cell would therefore be very beneficial to individuals with infection. In addition, Drew and colleagues (1983, 1984) discuss the presence of a factor in human milk, not found in colostrum, that is cytotoxic for human peripheral blood mononuclear cells and human lymphocytes from milk and colostrum. The role of this factor remains unknown but may be involved in protecting the infant against action of maternal lymphocytes in human milk. The phagocytic activity of polymorphonuclear leukocytes is also inhibited by a lipid or lipid-soluble fraction in human colostrum but not in mature milk (Pickering *et al.*, 1983).

Conclusions

The sections above review the functions and proposed mechanisms of action of anti-infective properties of human milk. The most obvious immunologic role of the mammary gland is supplying antibodies to the offspring. The other cellular and protein elements discussed appear to be functional, although the degree of their importance to the infant's health and the mechanisms by which they carry out their functions require further delineation. The benefits or hazards these immunologic components may have on the infant's health are considered in the following section.

Effects of Breast-Feeding on Infant Health

We are concerned with exploring all possible influences of infant feeding on morbidity, growth, and mortality during the first year of life. Since anti-infective factors in human milk are often cited in support of breast-feeding, we discuss its expected benefits and hazards in relation to these elements. How may these effects vary with the degree of supplementation? Can they be expected to persist after breast-feeding ceases?

Benefits of breast-feeding

Limited research data on anti-infective effects may be categorized by function:

* effect on gut environment
* effect on gut maturation and penetration of molecules
* protection against allergies
* effect on respiratory tract

Effect on gut environment

The predominant organism in the feces of breast-fed infants is *Lactobacillus bifidus*. A relationship between its presence among breast-fed infants and resistance to infection with specific types of *E. coli*, particularly those associated with infantile gastroenteritis has been suggested. The mechanism by which human milk confers this protection is unclear. Stools of breast-fed infants have higher counts of bifido-bacteria and are more acid than those of babies receiving cow's milk or formula. These gut characteristics may inhibit the growth of *E. coli*. See figure IV-5 for possible pathways involved in providing this protection.

Because the ideas in figure IV-5 stem from *in vitro* research primarily, whether these pathways may be functional *in vivo* should be questioned. Further investigation is necessary to determine if *L. bifidus* is itself a protective agent, or if human milk provides interacting substances that collectively provide this protection.

Stephens *et al*. (1984) investigated effects of antibody levels in breast-fed and bottle-fed infants from age six days to nine months. They found no differences between groups in tetanus toxoid vaccine response. Infants were vaccinated around the time of weaning which may account for this result. Evaluating this result on wholly breast-fed infants who have been antigenically stimulated with the vaccine would be useful. Interestingly, bottle-fed infants display higher concentrations of antibodies to *E. coli* "O" lipopolysaccharide antigens, perhaps because of their exposure to antigens

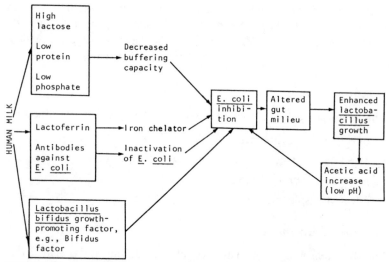

FIGURE IV-5   Effects of breast milk on gut environment.

other than those breast-fed babies experience or differences in gut environment.

Although we are cautious in applying conclusions from animal experiments to humans, it is necessary to consider them, since at this early stage in research, they allow hypothesis of mechanisms that may be functional in humans. For example, Pitt *et al.* (1977) demonstrated the importance of mononuclear phagocytes as protection against necrotizing enterocolitis in neonate rats consuming maternal milk. This may be an avenue worth pursuing in investigating necrotizing enterocolitis in humans.

A final point of interest is the altered susceptibility of infants to infection after immunization with attenuated polio virus. Warren *et al.* (1961), studying the influence of breast milk on intestinal infection with Sabin Type 1 polio virus vaccine, detected the virus in the feces of significantly fewer breast-fed than bottle-fed babies, indicating a possible inhibitory effect of milk on intestinal infection by the virus. Milk and sera from some mothers showed antibody activity specific for the virus, which was probably responsible for interfering with its establishment in the intestine.

Effect on gut maturation and penetration of molecules

The surface of the gastrointestinal tract forms the barrier between the interior of the organism and the molecules to which it is exposed. It therefore serves as a barrier to antigen absorption. In addition, its large number of lymphocytes and lymphatic vessels stresses its importance as an immunologic organ. The recognized digestive and absorptive function of the gastrointestinal tract across the mucosal surface in the neonate, and possibly all through infancy, is underdeveloped, especially in the premature infant. Factors present in human milk may facilitate maturation of the intestinal barrier and provide antibodies (especially sIgA) to exclude antigen at the surface (Walker, 1979), thereby protecting against infection or systemic/ atopic responses. It has been reported that sIgA is involved in protecting against permeability to antigens and microorganisms. Since active production of sIgA antibodies in intestinal secretions appears only after several months of intraluminal antigenic stimulus to local precursors of sIgA-producing plasma cells (Selner *et al.*, 1968), we speculate that sIgA in human colostrum and milk provides a passive mucosal barrier against penetration (Walker, 1973, as cited by Walker, 1979). Observations in animals such as the pig have suggested the presence of "trophic factors" in maternal milk that enhance maturation of the small intestine. These factors may be present in human colostrum and milk.

More recent research (Vukavić, 1984) suggests breast-feeding may not affect gut closure and consequent penetration of IgA into the circulation. Vukavić suggests that duration of gut permeability to macromolecules varies, with infants being either good or poor IgA absorbers. Vukavić used level of serum IgA as an index of postnatal macromolecular absorption and evaluated the influence of breast-feeding on gut closure. She failed to report the amount of colostrum the infants consumed; although difficult to monitor, it is an important variable that may also influence the serum IgA level. Further study is required to determine age of gut closure in humans and the effect of breast-feeding and other foods on it.

The quantity and immunochemistry of invading molecules is of concern when studying the phenomenon of immune responses and tolerance. Additional variables complicating the study of immune responses to antigen stimulation are the age at which exposure to food antigens occurs and the weaning process. Ferguson and Strobel (1984) investigated the ability of mice at various ages to respond to intragastric intubation of ovalbumin (OVA). Feeding OVA to adult mice produced tolerance, but not in week-old mice. Tolerance can be reestablished if feeding of OVA continues to day 14. This pattern changes when animals are fed OVA *during* the weaning period when they display no subsequent oral tolerance and a decreased suppression of cell-mediated immune response. At the time of weaning, there is also a loss of or lower intake of maternal milk, change in gut flora, and increased exposure to "new" food antigens. All of these could well account for the resistance to tolerance induction. This finding is of importance in human neonates since protein antigens encountered when the immune system and gut environment are immature may cause the infant to be sensitized to the antigen and consequently lead to immune responses to foods.

Protection against allergies

Low levels of IgA at birth and the immature gastrointestinal tract are of concern in terms of the infant's capacity to protect itself from a systemic immune response against ingested macromolecules.

A wholly breast-fed infant is protected from food allergies in two ways. First, the infant is not exposed to antigenic molecules of other foods. Second, human milk sIgA against a food allergen may alleviate a local or systemic response. Hanson *et al.* (1977) demonstrated lower levels of serum IgG antibodies to cow's milk proteins in infants on mixed feeding for several weeks compared to those weaned abruptly to cow's milk, indicating possible protection by human milk sIgA. After a period of mixed feeding, the infant's local antibody response probably develops slowly and becomes more efficient, thereby reducing the risk of developing allergy to food protein. This last finding has not been demonstrated in their more recent work (Fallström et al., 1984). The benefits of breast-feeding for an allergy-prone infant may be more pronounced, although further research on the topic is required.

On the other hand, the foods mothers consume, especially cow's milk, may initiate food allergies in their breast-fed infants (Gerrard and Shenassa, 1983a, b). The studies above should be interpreted with care since they do not allow one to deduct the percentage of breast-fed infants who develop allergies. It is assumed that only a handful of babies react to the trace amounts of antigen in their mother's milk—an IgE-mediated response. Allergies precipitated by the infants' consuming cow's milk are caused by exposure to large amounts of antigen and are probably not IgE-mediated.

Effect on respiratory tract

If human milk provides local protection, it is plausible to assume that these protective substances, especially IgA, line the mucosa of the oral cavity (especially the nasal pharyngeal area) and protect against infection. Hemagglutination-inhibition activity against influenza A in human milk has been documented, indicating that immunoglobulins directed against this antigen may be present. Downham and coworkers (1976) demonstrated IgA and IgA antibody to respiratory syncytial virus in 18 of 21 specimens of colostrum. They speculated that inhaled IgA provides this localized protection. Infants sometimes inhale milk, and regurgitate it through the nose.

Hazards of breast-feeding

Although maternal milk fulfills numerous protective functions, it is not without immunologic hazards. Breast milk of hepatitis B carrier mothers has been implicated as a possible cause of newborn infection. The infant could ingest infectious serum from cracked nipples, or the virus may be present in milk itself (Krugman, 1975). The antigen may also be transported transplacentally or during birth. Since hepatitis B antigen is found in milk, this may be an important mode of transmission, although further research is needed to clarify this point. On the other hand, Beasley et al. (1975) provided evidence against breast milk as a mode of vertical transfer of the antigen among Taiwanese mothers who carried it.

Although further studies are required, Kinoshita *et al.* (1984) found ATLV/HTLV antigen on cultured human milk mononuclear cells which may present a source of infection to infants. Their data are not conclusive for horizontal transmission of the virus but should be considered as indicating a possible hazard for infants breast-fed by mothers who are sero-positive for this virus (probably true for only a small percentage).

Breast-fed infants whose mothers have high amounts of antibodies to specific bacteria or viruses (e.g., diphtheria and tetanus) may not actively produce antibodies to immunization doses of these organisms because of the inhibitory activity of the milk immunoglobulins. The same effect may occur in prenatally transferred immunologic protection. Immunization may therefore be carried out at a later age or the infant should be reimmunized.

Further possible consequences of transfer of immunologic components from mother to infant are induction of tolerance, initiation of graft versus host disease, and initiation of hypersensitivity to foreign maternal antigens. These phenomena have been described in experiments in animals; their relevance to man is questionable (Beer and Billingham, 1975).

Persistence of effects after breast-feeding ceases

Since breast milk primarily provides local protection, we speculate that immunologic benefits persist for as long as the infant receives it. When breast-feeding ceases, it is possible for passively acquired immune elements to be present locally, although it is not known if this continues for any significant period of time. Secretory IgA lining the mucosa may persist when breast-feeding ceases. This immunoglobulin will therefore provide protection against infection until it is degraded or degenerates.

Relationship between degree of supplementation and immunologic protection

Little is known about how the degree of supplementation alters the benefits of breast-feeding. Probably all the immunologic benefits cited above are more pronounced in a wholly breast-fed infant than in one mixed fed. This situation may be because the wholly breast-fed infant consumes larger amounts of immune elements, while babies fed supplementary food have increased exposure to foreign antigens.

Other factors affecting neonate and infant health status

Factors such as nutritional status and exposure to pathogens are also important in maintaining optimal infant health conditions.

A wholly breast-fed infant is less exposed to pathogens that gain admittance via food, but is exposed to bacteria present on the breasts and on objects or persons it comes in contact with. On the other hand, a partially breast-fed infant, or one fed foods other than breast milk, is exposed to microorganisms that contaminate the raw food, water, and utensils used for cooking and feeding. This problem has greater significance in developing countries (Barrell and Rowland, 1980; Rowland et al., 1978; Surjono et al., 1980). Furthermore, preparing and storing supplemental foods under unsanitary conditions increases bacterial counts and the number of bacteria the infant ingests. The dose of pathogens ingested, the infant's immune status, and its nutritional status interact to determine the degree of illness and extent of complications. These other foods may also be of poor nutritional quality (Rowland et al., 1978).

Conclusions

A newborn appears capable of immune response. The capabilities of the immune system at birth reflect passive immunity acquired prenatally and presence of the functional elements of the immune system. At birth, on exposure to various antigenic materials and colonization of the gut, the immune system continues to develop. Dietary intake, nutritional status, and type of feeding (breast milk versus other foods) also influence the infant's ability to protect itself immunologically. Although prenatally acquired antibodies are expected to provide a level of protection after birth, the infant immune system is not as mature as the adult's. Additionally, the passively acquired antibodies are degraded over time. At four to six months of age, the level of immunoglobulins in the infant is low (table IV-2) and the baby may be more susceptible to infection at this time. Human milk provides the infant certain health benefits via consumption of protective (immune and other) factors which may be most essential during the four-to-six-month period and weaning.

A variety of cellular factors in human milk, such as B and T cells and macrophage and molecular factors, such as immunoglobulins and complement, provide protection against infection. These factors may act locally in the environment of the gastrointestinal and respiratory tracts by aiding in maturation of the former and fighting against allergies. Systemic effects may take place, although little evidence can be found.

Evidence suggests that human milk affects infant health in any of the following ways: (1) offering protection via consumption of antimicrobial factors, (2) limiting exposure to pathogens, and (3) providing better nutritional quality than other foods, especially in developing countries, thereby affecting immune status, nutritional status, morbidity, and growth. When breast-feeding ceases, continued protection of the infant against infection is doubtful. If these factors are acting locally and breast-feeding ends, it is logical to assume that they are no longer being ingested. Those immune factors that line the gastrointestinal and respiratory tract (e.g., immunoglobulins) continue to protect for as long as they are present, which depends on their half-life or degradation by enzymes. If the effects are systemic, a speculative notion because of lack of evidence, the benefits or effects on health may be long term. Finally, the effects on health are probably more pronounced in wholly breast-fed infants since they are consuming increased amounts of antimicrobial factors and have limited exposure to pathogens. Infants being fed other foods only will be exposed to increased amounts of pathogens compared to those partially breast-fed. With partial breast-feeding, some protection is provided via ingestion of some human milk, whereas an infant totally weaned from the breast is deprived of all the antimicrobial factors of human milk.

EPIDEMIOLOGICAL EVIDENCE

The immunological evidence summarized above provides biological bases to hypothesize a beneficial effect of breast-feeding on infant morbidity and mortality. Based on the immunological literature reviewed earlier in this chapter, it is reasonable to expect an association between breast-feeding and decreased morbidity and mortality. Observing such a relationship in humans would provide further evidence that the association may be causal. We discuss the methodological issues involved in observing and quantifying such an association and review epidemiologic studies in the context of these methodologic issues that include problems of selecting and measuring the outcome variable, control for confounding variables, sample size, research design, and temporality of events. The review of results asks questions aimed at characterizing specifically the relationship between infant feeding and morbidity and mortality.

Methodological Issues

Several recent articles focus on methodological problems of studies examining the relationship between breast-feeding and infant morbidity or mortality (Cunningham, 1981; Feachem and Koblinsky, 1984; Jason *et al.*, 1984; Kovar *et al.*, 1984; Millman, 1984; Sauls, 1979). Repeatedly discussed are problems in defining breast-feeding and study outcomes. Other methodological issues discussed include sample size problems, nonblind assessment of study results, inappropriate or insufficient statistical analysis, and the need to specify more detailed hypotheses.

Evaluating the effect of breast-feeding on infant morbidity and mortality presents challenges typical of many epidemiological research issues. Many authors focus on problems of measuring the effect of an exposure on an outcome in a setting where randomization is not feasible. Study design problems, defining the population at risk, identifying and assessing confounding, and temporality have received much attention in the epidemiological literature. Many texts are available to guide the researcher conducting epidemiological studies. The methodological problems cited in recent reviews can be managed by applying existing methodology developed to answer other research questions.

Studying the effect of breast-feeding on infant morbidity and mortality is in many ways easier than some other research questions epidemiologists have studied. Study populations are readily available because the exposures and outcomes are common events, the time between them is short, and new cohorts are accessible in various settings and circumstances. Below we consider methodological issues as they pertain to infant feeding and its effect on morbidity or mortality.

Definition of exposure and outcome variables

Variables must be defined and definitions described to the reader (see chapter 2). Here we mention some points regarding the outcome variable. The researcher's conceptualization of the biological mechanisms by which breast-feeding can affect morbidity and mortality and feasibility determine the choice of outcome variable.

Early studies chose such outcome variables as all mortality or all hospital admissions (Asher, 1952; Davis, 1913; Douglas, 1950; Howarth, 1905). In settings where infant mortality was primarily attributed to infectious causes, such outcome variables were appropriate. With increasing knowledge of the immunological properties of breast milk has come an attempt to focus studies on more specific outcomes – infections caused by specific pathogens (France *et al.*, 1980; Gunn *et al.*, 1979; Pullan *et al.*, 1980), and to link these studies to clinical and laboratory evidence of the immunological action of breast milk components on that pathogen. In developing hypotheses for the effect of breast-feeding on morbidity and mortality, it is important to consider the immunological evidence about particular pathogens and the mechanisms by which breast milk might act on them and on the course of illness. This latter point is relevant in comparing the effects of breast-feeding on gastrointestinal and respiratory infections.

After developing a hypothesis and choosing an outcome of interest, the operational definition of the outcome variable is greatly influenced by practical considerations. Data sources (hospital records, maternal recall) and resources (feasibility of collecting specimens) will influence the choice and definition of the outcome variable.

Confounding variables

As in all observational studies, the subjects in those reviewed here are preselected into exposure categories. The mothers chose the feeding method to which the infant subjects were exposed. Their decisions are associated with numerous variables which may also be independently associated with the study outcomes, including family socioeconomic status, maternal age and parity, birth weight and gestational age, delivery complications, and previous exposure to breast-feeding. The potential confounders may independently affect infant morbidity or mortality, but may also be associated with other variables affecting the infant's probability of becoming ill or dying from an illness. Such variables might include presence of piped water or a refrigerator, access to health care, and mother's ability to recognize symptoms or illness.

The interrelationships among the variables associated with mothers' feeding choices and the likelihood of infant illness or death have not been thoroughly conceptualized or described. Thus, studies which try to control for confounding often seem arbitrary in their choice of confounding variables. Decisions to consider a variable a potential confounder must be made in the design stage, based on the literature and conceptualization of the relationship between the potential confounder and the study exposure and outcome variables. The final decision to control for a variable must be based on sound epidemiologic criteria (Kleinbaum *et al.*, 1982). Recent studies using univariate or multivariate methods to control for independent variables have often not gone through the appropriate procedures or described the process of assessing confounding. It cannot be known whether the control for such variables removes existing biases in the measure of effect or introduces new ones.

Temporality

In any epidemiological study, it is essential to know that the exposure, here infant-feeding, precedes the outcome, illness or death. Several researchers have raised this issue (Butz *et al.*, 1984; Jason *et al.*, 1984; Kovar *et al.*, 1984; Sauls, 1979).

Categorizing infants into groups according to the feeding mode prior to onset of illness is important, especially in case-control studies, which identify cases after illness begins. Problems may arise if sick infants are switched from one feeding category to another. A second problem is that short breast-feeding duration may be a consequence of death rather than its cause. Prospective studies can be designed which clearly define (1) the population at risk, for example, excluding infants who die before ever being fed; (2) the entry criteria to the study; and (3) causes of death which may be related to feeding. Such is not the case in surveys where mothers are asked to recall feeding and mortality histories over their entire reproductive period, although some researchers have tried to compensate for design problems in their statistical analysis (Butz *et al.*, 1984).

Sample size

Overall sample size must be planned to allow appropriate statistical analysis with sufficient power for testing hypotheses at predesignated alpha levels; research reports must discuss these issues. Some studies with quite small sample sizes, perhaps 20 or fewer infants (Berger *et al.*, 1983; Myers *et al.*, 1984), are not always included in table IV-10.

A second issue is sample size availability in each exposure group. Within a given population and infant age group there is generally one dominant feeding mode. It may be difficult to find adequate numbers in the alternative feeding group. Studies in preindustrial settings often cannot identify many infants in the exclusively bottle-fed category, while studies in industrialized settings have not always elicited adequate numbers breast-fed exclusively for sufficient periods of time. Such situations may produce categorization schemes that ignore theoretical distinctions; as an example, in the Kanaaneh study (1972) exclusively and partially bottle-fed infants were placed in one category because only two babies had been exclusively bottle-fed. Measuring an effect beyond a certain age may be precluded, as in the United States where only 23 percent of women breast-feed for longer than five months (Martinez and Nalezienski, 1981). Since percentages breast-feeding exclusively through the fifth and sixth months are smaller, sample sizes are not readily available to test hypotheses about breast-feeding and its effect on morbidity at those ages and beyond.

Statistical analysis

The most glaring problems with statistical analysis are those of studies which do little or none of it, omitting even tests of significance. Statistical analysis is subject to various errors such as analyzing matched pair data which disregards the matching (Myers *et al.*, 1984; Pullan *et al.*, 1980).

Study design

Most of the studies reviewed use cohort (with prospective or retrospective data) or case-control design. In studying the effect of infant feeding on morbidity and mortality, it is relatively easy to identify a cohort and follow it prospectively or to reconstruct one. In either case, cohort study design allows one to deal with temporality and use survival analysis and related statistical techniques, particularly well-suited to measuring an effect of an exposure on a time-dependent outcome. The case-control study has problems in categorizing feeding after illness has started and possible biases introduced in the selection of cases and controls. Its advantage is in allowing the researcher greater ease in focusing on a particular disease outcome (Gunn *et al.*, 1979; Winberg and Wessner, 1971), and it may allow a more efficient use of resources.

Several studies combine features of several epidemiological designs— the cross-sectional survey and the reconstructed cohort (Butz *et al.*, 1984; Forman *et al.*, 1984; Goldberg *et al.*, 1984; Janowitz *et al.*, 1981). All were conducted in developing countries and used retrospective data on live births to women in their reproductive years. Some collected data on family living conditions at the time of each birth and at the time of interview. This method allows sample sizes in the range of one to five thousand births, although such a design has some objectionable qualities. Births occurring to a group of women aged 15 to 44 will have occurred over a 30-year period, raising questions about the mother's ability to provide accurate recall data and the comparability of the feeding, morbidity, and mortality experience. Most mothers in such settings provide information on more than one birth and all are included in the analysis; these are not truly independent observations and may present statistical problems. A final problem is that such groups of infants do not represent an actual cohort. If an infant's mother died or migrated before the upper limit of the study (usually 44), then that infant's feeding, morbidity, and mortality experience will not be included in the study. It is unclear what inferences can be made from such types of studies.

Review of Studies

For the general hypothesis that levels of morbidity and mortality decrease with increasing levels of breast-feeding, *levels of morbidity and mortality* refer to any morbidity or mortality of infectious origin, whether measured as total episodes per unit of time, or as time to first episode; *levels of breast-feeding* refer to any ordered categorization of breast-feeding by duration, degree of supplementation, or combination thereof, in which one group may be considered to have had more "exposure" to breast-feeding than the one to which it is compared.

Breast-feeding versus its alternatives: Effect on morbidity and mortality

Over 50 studies examining the relationship among breast-feeding, morbidity, and mortality are summarized in table IV-10. Conducted over the last 80 years, these studies represent varied cultural, economic, and historical settings. Relative risk (RR) estimates are those of the authors or calculated from the authors' data; they represent the magnitude and direction of the effect of *not* breast-feeding on morbidity and mortality.

Nearly all studies to date have found breast-feeding associated with lower morbidity and mortality from various causes. The exceptions are Adebonojo (1972), Cushing and Anderson (1982), Dugdale (1971), Fergusson *et al.*, (1978, 1981), Frank *et al.* (1982), Gurwith *et al.* (1981), Pullan *et al.* (1980), and Taylor *et al.* (1982). Of the studies with negative findings, only Dugdale's was conducted in a low-income country; the others were conducted in modern, industrialized nations such as the United States or England. The negative findings might be explained by the overall lower incidence of disease, requiring greater sample sizes to assure adequate power, or by

TABLE IV-10

Studies testing hypothesis that morbidity and mortality increase with decreasing breast-feeding by income areas

Study	Study Date & Site	N[1]	Study Design[2]	Feeding Groups[3]	Outcome Variable	Supports Hypothesis?[4]	Relative Risk[5] (RR)	Control Variables
HIGHER INCOME AREAS								
Howarth, 1905	1900–03 Derby, England	8343	Cohort	3	Mortality	+	2.83	None
Davis, 1913	1910–11 Boston, Mass., USA	2248a 736b	Case-control	2	Mortality	+	7.56	None
Woodbury, 1922	8 U.S. cities	22422	Cohort	3	Mortality	+	Range: 1.45– 8.43	None
Grulee et al., 1934	1924–29 Chicago, Ill., USA	20061	Cohort	3	Mortality Infections Respiratory infections GI infections	+ + + +	54.78 1.70 1.39 3.08	None
Deeny & Murdock, 1944	1941–42 Belfast, Ireland	554a 477b	Case-control	2	Mortality	+	2.88	Income, housing, birth order, domestic hygiene
Mayes, 1947	1945 Brooklyn, N.Y., USA	143	Cohort	2	Neonatal diarrhea Deaths from diarrhea	+	16.00 30.00	None

TABLE IV-10 (Continued)

Study	Study Date & Site	N^1	Study Design[2]	Feeding Groups[3]	Outcome Variable	Supports Hypothesis?[4]	Relative Risk[5] (RR)	Control Variables
HIGHER INCOME AREAS (continued)								
Douglas, 1950	1946–48 England	<4669[6]	Cohort	2	Deaths	+	1.73	Social class
					Hospitalizations for gastroenteritis & diarrhea	+	2.23	
					Diarrhea	?	1.07	
					Respiratory infections	+	1.20	
Robinson, 1951	1936–42 England	3708	Cohort	3	Mortality	+	5.62	Birth order
					Morbidity	+	2.57	
					Case fatality	+	2.17	
Naish, 1951	1940s England	100	Cohort	2	Morbidity	+	4.12	Social class
Asher, 1952	1949–50 Birmingham, Ala., USA	1044	Case-control	2	Hospitalizations for infection			None
					0–16 wks	+	4.71	
					5–16 wks	+	4.56	
Mann-heimer, 1955	1943–47 Stockholm, Sweden	634	Cohort	3	Mortality			None
					2 mos	+	1.49	
					3 mos	+	3.36	
					4–6 mos	+	3.57	
					7–9 mos	+	2.40	
					10–12 mos	+	1.27	

TABLE IV-10 (continued)

Study	Study Date & Site	N[1]	Study Design[2]	Feeding Groups[3]	Outcome Variable	Supports Hypothesis?[4]	Relative Risk[5] (RR)	Control Variables
HIGHER INCOME AREAS (continued)								
Yekutiel et al., 1958	1954 Israel	130	Cohort	4	Diarrhea	+	—	None
Winberg & Wessner, 1971	Goteberg, Sweden	99	Case-control	*	Neonatal septicemia	+	—	Clinic, birth wt, parity, gestational age
Adebonojo, 1972	Marin Co., Calif., USA	113	Cohort	2	Morbidity	—	—	None
Downham et al., 1976	1973–74 Newcastle, England	115a 167b	Case-control	2	Respiratory syncytial virus	+	5.08	Social class
Fergusson et al., 1978	New Zealand	1210	Cohort	4	Mortality Hospitalizations	— —	— —	Maternal education, marital status, living conditions
Chandra, 1979	Canada	60	Cohort	2	Respiratory infection / Otitis / Diarrhea / Dehydration / Pneumonia	+ / + / + / ? / ?	2.33 / 9.56 / 3.20 / — / —	SES, parental education, family size

TABLE IV-10 (continued)

Study	Study Date & Site	N[1]	Study Design[2]	Feeding Groups[3]	Outcome Variable	Supports Hypothesis?[4]	Relative Risk[5] (RR)	Control Variables
HIGHER INCOME AREAS (continued)								
Cunningham, 1979	1974–76 Cooperstown, N.Y., USA	503	Cohort	3	Morbidity	+	—	Paternal education, maternal age, birth order & wt, baby's sex
Fallot et al., 1980	1978 Onondaga Co., N.Y., USA	360	Case-control	3	Morbidity	+	3.44	Social class (clinic vs. private patients)
France et al., 1980	1977–78 Arkansas, USA	453	Cohort	2	Salmonella	+	96	Social class (clinic vs. private patients)
Pullan et al., 1980	1977–78 England	127a	Case-control	2	Respiratory syncytial virus	+	2.2	Baby's age, social class
		503b	Control			—	—	Maternal care & smoking, presence of other child in room
Fergusson et al., 1981	New Zealand	1156	Cohort	2	GI illness Respiratory infections	+ −	2–3 1	Sociodemographic variables & maternal smoking
Gurwith et al., 1981	1976–79 Canada	104	Cohort	2	Rotavirus infection	—	1.43	None

THE INFANT-FEEDING TRIAD

TABLE IV-10 (continued)

Study	Study Date & Site	N[1]	Study Design[2]	Feeding Groups[3]	Outcome Variable	Supports Hypothesis?[4]	Relative Risk[5] (RR)	Control Variables
HIGHER INCOME AREAS (continued)								
Cushing & Anderson, 1982	1979 N. Mexico, USA	40	Cohort	2	Diarrhea	–	N.A.	
Dagan & Pridan, 1982	1978 Israel	480a 502b	Case-control	2	ER Morbidity Clinic visits	+ +	11.7 36.4	Residence, maternal education, social class None
Frank et al., 1982	1976–80 Texas, USA	81	Cohort	2	Respiratory infections	–	—	Maternal age, smoking, SES; baby's sex, birth rank
Taylor et al., 1982	1975 England	13,135	Cohort	*	Morbidity	–	—	
Myers et al., 1984	1979–80 Iowa, USA	20	Cohort	2	Respiratory infections GI illnesses	– +	— —	Baby's birth wt, age, sex

TABLE IV-10 (continued)

Study	Study Date & Site	N[1]	Study Design[2]	Feeding Groups[3]	Outcome Variable	Supports Hypothesis?[4]	Relative Risk[5] (RR)	Control Variables
LOWER INCOME AREAS								
Welbourn, 1958	1950–55 Uganda	1394	Cohort	2	GI infection Respiratory infection	+ +	3.33 1.80	None
French, 1967	1958–60 Navaho Indians, USA	139	Cohort	2	Morbidity 0–3 mos 4–6 mos 7–9 mos 10–12 mos 13–15 mos	 + + + + –	 8.24 ** 16.20 3.00 .38	None
McKenzie et al., 1967	1962–63 Jamaica	204a	Case-control	4	Mortality	–	.55	Age & sex
Wray & Aguirre, 1969	1963–64 Colombia	119	C-S/S	3	Diarrhea 0–5 mos 6–11 mos	 + +	 2.91 1.64	None
Dugdale, 1971	1960–65 Kuala Lumpur	250	Cohort	*	Respiratory & alimentary illnesses	–	—	Ethnicity, baby's sex, family income & size
Schaefer, 1971	1965–66 Eskimos, Alaska, USA	469	Case-control	2	Otitis media	+	13.4	Settlement (degree of urbanization)

TABLE IV-10 (continued)

Study	Study Date & Site	N[1]	Study Design[2]	Feeding Groups[3]	Outcome Variable	Supports Hypothesis?[4]	Relative Risk[5] (RR)	Control Variables
LOWER INCOME AREAS (continued)								
Kanaaneh, 1972	1971 Arab villages in Israel	610	Cohort	4	Mortality			None
					> 6 mos vs. < 6 mos	+	24.77	
					> 3 mos vs. < 3 mos	+	6.97	
Plank & Milanesi, 1973	1969–70 Chile	1712	Cohort	3	Mortality			None
					1 mo	+	2.07	
					3 mos	+	2.80	
					6 mos	+	1.99	
Chandra, 1979	1979 India	70	Cohort	2	Respiratory infections	+	1.91	SES, parental education, occupation, family size
					Otitis	+	2.48	
					Diarrhea	+	3.01	
					Dehydration	+	4.67	
					Pneumonia	+	4.00	
Gunn et al., 1979	1978 Bahrain	42a 42b	Case-control	2	Cholera	+	9.0	Baby's age, residence
Maynard & Hammes, 1979	1960–62 Alaska, USA	322	Cohort	2	Morbidity	+	1.40	None

TABLE IV-10 (continued)

Study	Study Date & Site	N^1	Study Design[2]	Feeding Groups[3]	Outcome Variable	Supports Hypothesis?[4]	Relative Risk[5] (RR)	Control Variables
LOWER INCOME AREAS (continued)								
Janowitz et al., 1981	1977–78 Egypt	2907	C-S/S	*	Mortality	+	—	Maternal education
Lepage et al., 1981	1977–78 Rwanda	2339	Cohort	2	Mortality	+	1.9	None
Clavano, 1982	1973–77 Philippines	9886	Cohort	3	Sepsis Oral thrush Diarrhea	+ + +	72 77 51	None
Mittal et al., 1983	India	148a 42b	Case-control	2	Diarrhea	+	2.55	Age, SES
Butz et al., 1984	1976–77 Malaysia	5573	C-S/S	*	Mortality	+	—	Having piped water, toilet facilities; ethnicity, maternal age & education, pregnancy interval, previous stillbirths, no. of persons in household, income, birthplace, rurality, baby's birth year

TABLE IV-10 (continued)

Study	Study Date & Site	N^1	Study Design[2]	Feeding Groups[3]	Outcome Variable	Supports Hypothesis?[4]	Relative Risk[5] (RR)	Control Variables
LOWER INCOME AREAS (continued)								
Forman et al., 1984	1978 Pima Indians, Arizona, USA	832	C-S/S	5	GI illness	+	1.5	Season, baby's age, birth year, SES
Goldberg et al., 1984	1980 Brazil	3457	C-S/S	2	Mortality	+	1.85	Residence, education, employment, parity, maternal age at last birth, birth interval, health services use

Notes: 1. Number = total sample size unless otherwise noted; a = cases; b= controls; 2. C-S/S = cross-sectional or survey; 3. When only 2 feeding groups were studied, the contrast may be exclusively and partially breast-fed or to partially breast-fed and nonbreast-fed; 4. Conclusions are summarized as supporting (+), not supporting (−), or inconclusive (?) in relation to hypothesis, based on tests of significance, measures of effect (RR), or other statistics; 5. Relative risk (RR) was calculated from data on morbidity or mortality incidence in the exposed category (nonbreast-feeding) divided by incidence in the nonexposed category (breast-feeding). With case-control data, the odds ratio is calculated as an estimate of RR. In comparing 3 or more groups, the 2 furthest ends of the continuum are contrasted (nonbreast-fed to exclusively breast-fed). A dash (—) = RRs unavailable or could not be calculated from the author's data; 6. Exclusions from sample made, but author does not give number (*) continuous variable (**) 0 in breast-feeding cell.

a lower relative effect because of the availability of hygienic, properly prepared breast milk alternatives. In studies which observe an effect, risk of illness or death is at least doubled for the nonbreast-fed infant compared to the breast-fed.

Does the effect persist after control for confounding?

As indicated, few studies examining the relationship between breast-feeding and morbidity try to control for extraneous variables. Those that do, stratify, match, and restrict as the most common methods to control for variables thought to be confounders; some use multivariate analysis.

Two studies used multivariate analysis to control for confounding. Dugdale (1971) controlled for ethnicity, infant's sex, family income and size; he found no association between duration of breast-feeding and respiratory or alimentary illnesses in 250 infants in Kuala Lumpur. Fergusson *et al.* (1978), who controlled for maternal education, single versus two-parent homes, and living conditions, found no association between breast-feeding and mortality and hospitalizations, but an association with number of medical consultations and symptoms in 1,156 infants in New Zealand. After following the same group through age two and controlling for various sociodemographic variables and maternal smoking, Fergusson *et al.* (1981) found a two- to threefold effect of breast-feeding on gastrointestinal illness but not on respiratory illness. Taylor *et al.* (1982) found no effect of breast-feeding on morbidity for 13 thousand babies in England after controlling for maternal age and smoking, infant's sex and birth rank, and socioeconomic status. Pullan *et al.* (1980) found a twofold effect on respiratory syncytial virus in England after controlling for infant's age and social class, but none after additional control for maternal care and smoking and presence of another child in the baby's room at night.

Remaining studies which controlled for more than one extraneous variable found a breast-feeding effect. In their Malaysian survey, Butz *et al.* (1984) used multivariate techniques to control for income, household size, rurality, year of infant's birth; maternal age, ethnicity, and education; and presence of piped water and toilet facilities. Goldberg *et al.* (1984) also used multivariate techniques in their Brazilian survey to control for residence, interval since last birth, use of maternal and child health services, and mother's education, employment, parity, and age at last birth. Forman and colleagues (1984) found an effect of breast-feeding on gastrointestinal illnesses among Pima Indians in Arizona after controlling for season, age of infection, birth year, and socioeconomic status. Studies by Dagan and

Pridan (1982), Gunn *et al.* (1979), and Mittal *et al.* (1983) all observed effects after controlling for two or three of these variables: social class, residence, maternal education, birth weight, infant's age or sex. Chandra (1979) matched infants according to socioeconomic status, parental education, and family size, finding significant associations between breast-feeding and lower levels of respiratory infections, otitis media, and diarrhea in Canada and India. Winberg and Wessner (1971) matched children as to clinic, birth weight, mother's age and parity, restricting on decision to breast-feed, birth weight, and maturity of newborn, and found a significant association between amount of breast milk intake in the first postpartum days and infections occurring four to ten days postpartum.

The remaining studies we reviewed which controlled for confounding did so for one variable only. Nonetheless, examining these studies and their conclusions is worthwhile. Several attempt to control for socioeconomic status (SES) or a proxy variable for it.

SES may be reasonably considered a major potential confounder; it is strongly associated with infant-feeding choices, as well as with infant morbidity and mortality. Studies using univariate approaches to control for SES are summarized in table IV-11; breast-feeding persists across strata in all of them. Social class differences do not fully explain the differences

TABLE IV-11

Relative risk (RR) of morbidity or mortality among nonbreast-fed infants by socioeconomic status (SES)

		Socioeconomic Status			
Study	Crude RR	Low	Middle	High	Variable
Deeny & Murdock, 1944	2.88	3.26	2.50	3.27	Income
Mannheimer, 1955	2.30	2.02	2.19	3.76	Income
Fallot *et al.*, 1980	3.44	1.67	—	3.84	Health care source
France *et al.*, 1980	96.00	a	—	76.00	Health care source
Downham *et al.*, 1976	5.08	2.79	5.61	8.88	Social class
Cunningham, 1979	—	1.84	—	1.81	Education

Notes: Variables in final column used as proxies for SES. Private patients assumed to be higher SES, clinic patients to be lower SES.
a = 0 cases in breast-feeding cell; RR cannot be calculated;
— = Data unavailable

observed in morbidity and mortality among breast-fed and nonbreast-fed infants. There is a clear need for further study on this matter.

Many researchers have been aware of the need to control for the infant's condition at birth, assuming that low birth weight, premature, or otherwise weak infants will be less likely to be breast-fed and more likely to experience morbidity and mortality. Birth weight has been used as the indicator of the infant's condition. Most studies controlled for birth weights by restricting the study population, matching, or by stratified analysis. Mannheimer's (1955) data show a benefit of breast-feeding to infants with birth weights greater than 2500 g. Other studies which match or restrict their samples to certain birth weights (Cunningham, 1979; Winberg and Wessner, 1971), also showed beneficial effects of breast-feeding after the effect of birth weight was controlled for. Conclusions of several studies (e.g., Clavano, 1982) would probably have been significantly altered had birth weight been controlled for.

How do effects of breast-feeding vary with infant's age?

It is appropriate to categorize infants of a given age by feeding practices, ignoring duration, when setting up categories, and evaluate morbidity or mortality within age-group intervals. Several studies take such an approach (see table IV-12). The beneficial effect of breast-feeding appears to peak between three to nine months and decline thereafter (French, 1967; Mannheimer, 1955; Woodbury, 1922), although Cunningham (1979) found the greatest benefit to be in the first two months of life. The data of W. H. Davis (1913), Deeny and Murdock (1944), and Plank and Milanesi (1973) show no obvious trend.

Future studies can apply the statistical technique of survival analysis, perfectly suited to allow calculation of the probability of an infant's becoming ill or dying within a given age interval—assuming it survives to that interval. When planning to use such analysis, a decision must be made about infants who switch from one feeding group to another, usually from breast-fed to nonbreast-fed. These infants can be dropped from the analysis after the interval when the feeding has changed, or they can be reassigned to a different feeding group in the interval after feeding has changed.

How does the effect vary with the degree of supplementation?

Because of methodological limitations discussed throughout this book, and inconsistency of results among studies, it is difficult to predict the effect

TABLE IV-12

Relative risk (RR) of morbidity or mortality among nonbreast-fed infants by age

Infant's Age (months)	Study & Date						
	Davis 1913	Woodbury 1922	Deeny & Murdock 1944	Mannheimer 1955	French 1967	Plank & Milanesi 1973	Cunningham 1979
0–1	} 8.00	3.24	2.88	—		2.07	} 6.34
1–2		4.24	3.56	1.49	8.24	—	
2–3		5.73	3.16	3.36		2.80	} 2.02
3–4		5.65	2.60			—	
4–5	} 9.17	5.48	—	} 3.57		—	} 2.76
5–6		8.43	—		a	1.99	
6–7	} 4.73	7.42	—	} 2.40		—	} 1.10
7–8		3.90	—		16.24	—	
8–9		3.34	—			—	
9–10	} 5.68	2.45	—	} 1.27		—	} 1.52
10–11		2.50	—		3.60	—	
11–12		1.45	—			—	} 1.66

a = 0 cases in breast-feeding cell; — = Data not available, RR cannot be calculated of differing degrees of supplementation on an infant at a given age, and the change in risk of disease over time. One would like to see, at a given age, a dose-response or threshold relationship between completeness of breast-feeding, or degree of supplementation, and level of morbidity and mortality among that age group.

The relationship should also be documented as it changes with the infant's age. In quantifying the relationship between supplementation and morbidity or mortality, defining the mixed category becomes crucial. It may be helpful to categorize the mixed group at a more detailed level, by exact number of feedings or by percentage of nutrient intake.

To study the effect of different levels of supplementation on morbidity and mortality, it is again desirable to categorize infants in each age group by degree of supplementation, observe morbidity and mortality, and re-categorize infants at successive age intervals. Three studies (Mannheimer, 1955; Plank and Milanesi, 1973; and Woodbury, 1922) have taken such an approach. Each compared mortality among three feeding groups (breast-fed, mixed fed, and artifically fed), and showed different relationships between supplementation and mortality levels. Woodbury (1922) showed that at each age to eight months in the U.S., the mixed feeding group experienced mortality between that of the breast-fed and artifically fed groups. Plank and Milanesi (1973) found mortality in rural Chile in the mixed fed group to be almost as high as among the artifically fed. See figure IV-6. In Mannheimer's study (1955) the mixed fed group had the lowest mortality, until six months, when the mixed and breast-fed groups experienced similar mortality levels.

Figure IV-7 summarizes several studies of breast, mixed, and artificial feeding compared to morbidity or mortality in each feeding category. Unfortunately, categories often reflected relative durations of breast-feeding, rather than completeness at a given age. This issue will be discussed further. The studies show a gradient of mortality and morbidity that increases as breast-feeding decreases; whether this reflects the effect of breast-feeding duration or supplementation is not clear.

One may conclude that at a given age within the first six months, infants in the fully breast-fed category appear to have a lower risk of morbidity than those in the nonbreast-fed (never breast-fed) category, but further detail is not readily available.

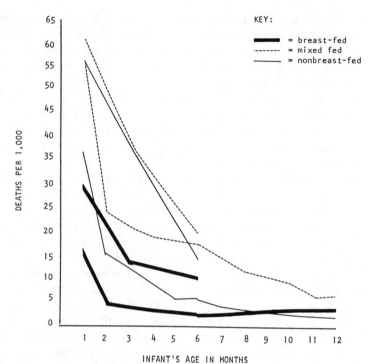

FIGURE IV-6 Mortality levels of breast-feeding and infant's age. Source: Data for rural Chile, 1969–1970, for ages 1–6 months come from Plank and Milanesi, 1973; data for United States, c. 1922, for ages 1–12 months come from Woodbury, 1922.

*How does duration of breast-feeding relate
to overall morbidity and mortality?*

Categorization schemes used often do not allow separation of supplementation and duration. In the Kanaaneh (1972) study in which categories reflected duration and degree of supplementation, number of hospitalizations increased with decreasing duration of breast-feeding and greater levels of supplementation, but there was no attempt to consider duration and supplementation separately.

Several studies related breast-feeding duration to overall morbidity during the first year of life. Some studies treat breast-feeding as a continuous variable reflecting the number of weeks or months during which the infant drank breast milk. Taylor and colleagues (1982) found no effect of breast-feeding duration on overall morbidity for a cohort of 13 thousand infants in England. The surveys of Janowitz *et al.* (1981) and Butz *et al.* (1984) observed an effect of breast-feeding duration on mortality in Egypt and Malaysia. Two studies categorized breast-feeding according to duration and considered effects on overall morbidity. Douglas (1950) found no significant difference in episodes of diarrhea among infants compared by duration of breast-feeding, but an inverse relationship between breast-feeding duration and lower respiratory infections. Cunningham (1979) categorized three groups by duration of breast-feeding (greater than 4.5 months, 6 weeks to less than 4.5 months, and less than 6 weeks) and found number of episodes of morbidity per year decreased with increasing duration of breast-feeding.

Does the effect of breast-feeding persist after breast-feeding ceases? This question is difficult to answer for several reasons. Questions discussed above have not been resolved, making it difficult to formulate and test specific hypotheses. The age of weaning and its duration vary greatly, further complicating efforts to evaluate possible long-term benefits of breast-feeding or a hypothesized systemic effect after breast-feeding has ceased. The association of morbidity with the weaning period may also obscure observation of a benefit of breast-feeding after weaning.

If the breast-fed infant is healthier at a given age than the nonbreast-fed infant, it is reasonable to assume that the healthier infant will maintain that advantage. It is less clear what benefits having been breast-fed will confer on the healthy infant in subsequent months. Researchers have not compared equally healthy populations of infants with different breast-feeding histories to examine subsequent patterns of morbidity and mortality.

The effect of other foods on morbidity and mortality.

No other food besides breast milk provides the infant with the immunological components discussed above. Thus the greatest contrast in morbidity and mortality would be expected between breast-fed and nonbreast-fed infants, yet, it is worthwhile to consider possible effects on morbidity and mortality resulting from particular choices of other foods. Other foods may differentially affect infant morbidity and mortality by exposing the infant to different levels of pathogens or by affecting nutritional status.

A few authors have contrasted breast milk alternatives themselves as well as contrasting breast milk with other foods. Yekutiel *et al.* (1958) found higher duration of diarrhea in infants aged one to two fed milk powder compared to a similar group fed fresh milk. Howarth (1905) looked at the following diets fed to 1,600 infants: milk and water, condensed milk, patent foods A, B, C, and D (presumably commercially prepared mixtures). He found death rates varying from 134/1,000 (patent food C) to 255/1,000 (condensed milk).

Categorizing the feeding variable in morbidity and mortality studies becomes more complex and crucial as diets become more varied and diverse. A categorization scheme needs to be developed that can be generalized to a variety of settings and take into consideration a specific hypothesis, for example, that storage methods or types of food which promote bacterial growth will lead to higher levels of morbidity and mortality. Preferably categorization schemes must be consistent across studies to allow comparison of results. Confounding variables must be controlled for, particularly those strongly associated with choice and preparation of foods.

The main factor preventing comparison of breast milk alternatives with each other has been lack of clearly defined, specific hypotheses, and of meaningful categorization schemes. Some differences in morbidity and mortality because of differences in pathogen levels and effects on nutritional status may be expected; further research is needed.

CONCLUSIONS

After the immunological and epidemiological evidence regarding the relationship among infant feeding, morbidity, and mortality have been separately evaluated, it is worthwhile to compare conclusions, be aware of areas of consensus, and point out areas for further research. Table IV-13

TABLE IV-13

Infant feeding, morbidity, and mortality:
Immunological and epidemiological evidence

Hypothesis	Immunological Evidence	Epidemiological Evidence
That breast-feeding protects infant from infection	Presence of antimicrobial factors in human milk and their viability (proven primarily in vitro) lets us expect breast-fed infants to be more likely to withstand infection and its complications than nonbreast-fed.	Most studies find nonbreast-fed infant at twice as likely to be sick or die than breast-fed infants.
That the effect changes with infant's age	Peak benefit may be expected between age 4–6 months.	Some studies show peak benefit between 3–9 months; inconsistent finding.
That the effect varies with degree of supplementation in a linear manner	Ingesting increased amount of breast milk may lead to increased levels of protection against disease. Simultaneously decreased ingestion of other foods may lead to decreased exposure to pathogens and lower risk of infection. Thus we expect a dose-response effect.	Only 3 studies examine this question using proper categorization schemes; study results inconsistent.
That breast-feeding duration is related to morbidity and mortality levels	We expect protective effect to persist as long as breast-feeding continues.	Studies inadequately separate duration from supplementation issues.
That the effect persists after breast-feeding ceases	Based on available evidence, no reason to expect effect after breast-feeding ceases.	No study properly examines this question.
Morbidity and mortality vary with choice of other foods	Other foods may affect morbidity and mortality levels through effects on nutritional status and variation in exposure to pathogens. No reason to expect independent effect of other foods on immune status.	Some variation but no consistent trend, no general categorization scheme, inadequate sample sizes.

summarizes the immunological and epidemiological evidence supporting six hypotheses. The first, that breast-feeding provides protection against infection, appears to be supported by a large body of laboratory and field evidence. Immunological studies have shown that infants receive a variety of components in breast milk which may provide direct protection against infection and may promote a gut environment more capable of resisting infection. The expected protective effect has been consistently observed in the majority of epidemiological studies conducted in a wide range of settings, over almost 80 years, in a variety of methodologies and study designs, with nonbreast-fed infants generally experiencing twice as much morbidity or mortality as breast-fed infants. In light of the large body of laboratory evidence and observation of the protective benefit of breast-feeding, it seems reasonable to assume that the effect exists, and should be further characterized.

Does the beneficial effect vary with the infant's age? Knowledge of the development of the infant's immune capacities suggests that the infant is especially vulnerable between four and six months of age, because of a decline in serum concentration of immunoglobulins. Several epidemiologic studies observed a peak benefit of breast-feeding between three and nine months of age; other studies find differing patterns or no discernible trend. In general, epidemiological studies have not been designed to test this hypothesis, and most do not allow such a comparison. Further research in this area should be conducted. Immunological research should examine in greater detail the development of the infant's immune system. More accurate techniques of measuring antimicrobial components in breast milk are needed to quantify in greater detail changes in them over time. This research should follow groups of mothers longitudinally to measure the degree of variation among individuals as well as populations.

Epidemiologic studies have been inadequate to test the hypotheses that the beneficial effect of breast-feeding is inversely related to degree of supplementation and persists as long as breast-feeding continues. One may expect a dose-response of breast-feeding on morbidity and mortality because varying degrees of supplementation simultaneously affect the dose of active immunological components the infant receives and the dose of pathogens it may be exposed to. When studying the effect of supplementation on the infant's probability of developing an infection or dying, it may be difficult to separate the two effects of immunoglobulin and pathogen exposure. In either case, one expects a dose-response of supplementation on the study outcomes. Categorization schemes have generally not separated duration from supplementation, preventing separate evaluation of each issue. Further epidemiologic research is needed in this area, particularly to develop appropriate categorization schemes and research designs, and to test these hypotheses.

The immunological evidence suggests that the immunological benefits of breast-feeding are local and confined to the period during which the immunological cells and molecules are active and present in the infant's system. Breast-feeding is unlikely to confer immunological protection after weaning. Epidemiologic studies have not been designed to examine this question.

Although other foods may alter the infant's nutritional status and level of exposure to pathogens, there is no reason to expect a direct effect of other foods on immune status. Because breast-feeding may also affect nutritional status and decreases exposure to pathogens, the greatest contrast in morbidity and mortality in any epidemiologic study would be expected to be between breast-fed and nonbreast-fed infants. The effect of other foods would probably be smaller. This fact must be considered when designing such a study, planning sample sizes, and selecting the sample. There is further need to develop a categorization scheme, suited to specific hypotheses regarding the effect of other foods on morbidity and mortality, and generalizable to a variety of research settings. Epidemiologic studies to date have not considered such issues, although they indicate variation in levels of morbidity and mortality with the choice of other foods.

5
INFANT FEEDING AND GROWTH

Considering the effect of infant foods on growth poses several methodological problems. In discussing morbidity and mortality, outcomes can be ranged on a continuum from positive to negative. With growth, positive outcomes are generally in the center of a continuum with negative extremes. Weight can increase or decrease although height is not lost. Thus the choice of standards—whether dietary recommendations, biochemical indicators, or growth—becomes crucial. Standards may have been developed in particular situations that may decrease their validity as research instruments. For example, dietary recommendations are often based on diets of breast-fed infants considered to be growing well. Growth standards in turn, have been based on norms of specific infant populations fed particular diets. In many studies a standard based on infants fed a particular diet is used to evaluate different infant diets. Present standards should be used with an awareness of their limitations. The issue of standards is an important area for further research.

Composition and quantity also complicate measurement of the effect of infant foods on growth. Studies comparing breast milk and formulas with different nutrient content and composition do not consider the total amount of nutrients the infant ingests in a given time. Thus it is important not only to compare nutrient content of similar volumes of different infant foods, but also volumes consumed and total nutrient intake compared to infant needs. These methodological issues have prevented feeding and growth studies from being as conclusive as those on feeding, morbidity, and mortality.

BIOLOGICAL EVIDENCE

Quantity of Nutrients

Nutrient requirements

Organizations in a number of countries have developed recommendations for infant nutrient intakes. Most commonly used are those of the World Health Organization (WHO) (Passmore *et al.*, 1974) and the National Academy of Sciences (NAS), National Research Council (NRC) (1980). Because methodological and ethical issues limit the extent of research on actual metabolic needs of infants, most recommendations are based on observed intakes of healthy infants. Studies on which these recommendations are based are fraught with problems of accurately measuring intakes, especially of breast milk, and evaluating growth (see below). Satisfactory health and growth of the reference infants indicate only that actual nutrient requirements are no greater than the amounts they are ingesting, but could be lower.

Current infant dietary recommendations apply only to healthy, full-term infants who have an adequate level of nutrient stores from their intrauterine endowment, immunologic protection, and relative maturity of other organs and biochemical systems (NRC, 1980; Passmore *et al.*, 1974). Infant nutrient stores are determined by maternal nutritional status (Eastman and Jackson, 1968; NRC, 1970), infant birth weight, gestational age (AAP, 1979), and health history. If a baby's nutrient stores are inadequate, if it suffers from chronic or acute infection, or was born prematurely or with a low weight, nutritional recommendations must be adjusted.

Infants need energy for maintenance, growth, and physical activity. On a body weight basis, maintenance needs are by far the largest component, declining slowly with age. The energy requirement for growth is higher in the first month of life but on a per kilogram basis declines rapidly thereafter. There is little information on energy requirements for physical activity in the infant.

A few studies have tried to determine infant metabolic requirements for energy; see table V-1 for their results compared with WHO and NAS recommendations. Energy requirements calculated by Waterlow and Thomson (1979) are somewhat lower than those developed by either WHO or NAS. These authors estimated energy needs for maintenance and growth on information from previous metabolic studies, making no allowance for

TABLE V-1

Infants' Energy Requirements (in kcal/kg)—results of several studies

Study	Age (months)							Underlying Assumptions/ Calculations
	0	1	2	3	4	5	6	
Passmore et al., 1974	120 ——————— 115 ——————— 110							Based on observed intakes of breast-fed infants
NRC, 1980	115 ———————————————— 105							Based on observed intakes of (presumably breast- & bottle-fed) infants
Waterlow & Thomson, 1979	122	114	105	102	99	90		Maintenance—82 kcal/kg Growth—along 25th %ile NAS standards; 5 kcal/g weight gained Physical activity—not included
Waterlow & Thomson, 1979, revised according to Foman, 1967	116	110	100	98	90	90		Same as above except composition of weight gain according to Fomon (1967)
Whitehead & Paul, 1981		104	97	91	89	87		Predicted growth along 50th %ile from regression equation of longitudinal data on intake, weight, & weight gain of healthy British breast-fed boys

the energy cost of physical activity. Maintenance requirements were based on a study of 8- to 18-month-old, hospitalized infants recovering from malnutrition. It is not known if these figures are applicable to younger or healthy infants. Waterlow and Thomson considered rate of growth along the 25th percentile desirable. There is no general consensus on "normal" or "optimal" growth in the Third World. The Waterlow and Thomson calculations assume a certain body composition of weight gain in terms of fat and protein. Introducing Fomon's (1967) data on body composition to Waterlow and Thomson's calculations gives a somewhat lower energy requirement (see table V-1). A later study by Whitehead and Paul (1981), using a regression equation to predict energy requirements, gave results lower even than Waterlow and Thomson's, although the presumed growth rate was at the 50th percentile.

Based on these few studies, current WHO and NAS recommendations for energy appear somewhat higher than actual requirements. However, much more careful research needs to be conducted on infant nutritional requirements before any firm conclusions can be drawn.

Although current recommendations for infant protein intake are based on observations of healthy infants (NRC, 1980; Passmore *et al.*, 1974), some research has been conducted on infants' biological needs for protein. Dietary protein is needed to replace losses from normal, continuing biological processes (maintenance) and to build new tissue for growth. Recommendations are usually based on mean values of individual intakes or requirements, plus a margin of safety usually equivalent to two standard deviations above the mean. Resulting recommendations should be high enough to cover actual requirements of most infants. While current WHO and NAS recommendations include this safety margin, some studies on biological needs do not, making it difficult to compare results.

Table V-2 shows results of several studies on protein requirements for infant growth and tissue maintenance. Only one study (Fomon, 1974) included a margin of safety and can be compared directly with WHO or NAS recommendations. Fomon's recommended protein intake is similar to the official recommendations. His results indicated that the protein requirement is no greater than 2.2 g/kg for infants zero to four months old, 2.0 g/kg from four to six months, but it could be lower.

Two other studies arrived at protein requirements somewhat lower than current WHO or NAS recommendations, since they did not provide a margin of safety. These few studies indicate that WHO and NAS protein recommendations are in close agreement with biological needs when a margin of safety is incorporated to account for variation in individual requirements.

Table V-3 gives requirements for other nutrients, for the most part, based on nutrient content of the quantity of breast milk consumed by infants without deficiency signs. An exception is the recommendation for vitamin D—in excess of the amount in breast milk and about four times the amount necessary to prevent rickets—made to improve calcium absorption and increase growth (NRC, 1980). Riboflavin requirements are based on energy requirements, and the requirement for vitamin B_6 (not included in the WHO recommendations) is based on the amount necessary to avoid deficiency symptoms in infants. Differences in the WHO and NAS recommendations result from different interpretations of previous research and differences in environmental conditions in areas in which the respective recommendations will be used.

TABLE V-2

Infants' protein requirements (in g of protein/kg unless otherwise stated)—
results of several studies

Study	Age (months) 0	1	2	3	4	5	6	Margin of Safety	Underlying Assumptions
Passmore et al., 1974	2.4[a] ———			1.85[a]	———		1.62[a]	2 standard deviations	Based on observed intakes of breast-fed infants
NRC, 1980	2.2[a] ———————						2.0[b]	2 standard deviations	Based on observed intakes of (presumably breast- & bottle-fed) infants
Fomon & May, 1958	1.875[a]	1.69[a]	1.53[a]	1.38[a]	1.22[a]		1.04[a]	None	Based on nitrogen retention studies maintenance requirement of 120 mg nitrogen/kg
Fomon, 1974	1.9 g/100 kcal[a]——1.7 g/100 kcal[a]—— (=2.2 g/kg) – (=2.0 g/kg) – (=1.8 g/kg)							Mean + 20%	Feeding trial with 1.62 g protein/100 kcal (0–4 mos); 1.4 g protein/100 kcal (4–12 mos)
Waterlow & Thomson, 1979	1.98	1.79	1.63	1.56	1.47		1.38	None	Maintenance: 120 mg nitrogen/kg; growth; along 25th %ile, NAS standards

[a] as egg or milk protein
[b] as mixed protein with 75 percent utilization efficiency

Meeting infant nutrient requirements

Fulfilling the increasing nutrient needs of a growing infant requires increasing amounts of food. Providing ever-increasing amounts of special infant foods is not always feasible, especially in the Third World. A family may not be able to purchase increasing quantities of commercial infant foods and a lactating woman may not be able to produce increasing quantities

TABLE V-3

Infants' vitamin and mineral requirements

Requirements	National Academy of Sciences		World Health Organization
	0−6 mos	6−12 mos	0−12 mos
Vitamin A (μg)	400.0	420.0	300.0
Vitamin D (μg)	10.0	10.0	10.0
Thiamin (mg)	0.5	0.3	0.3
Riboflavin (mg)	0.6	0.4	0.5
Niacin (mg)	8.0	6.0	5.4
Folic acid (μg)	45.0	30.0	60.0
Vitamin B$_6$ (mg)	0.6	0.3	NA
Vitamin B$_{12}$ (μg)	1.5	0.5	0.3
Vitamin C (mg)	35.0	35.0	20.0
Iron (mg)	15.0	10.0	5−10.0
Calcium (mg)	540.0	350.0	500−600.0

Sources: NRC, 1980; Passmore et al., 1974

of breast milk. How long can an infant be sustained exclusively on a particular special infant food, breast milk, commercial formula, or other milks, and when should the milk-based diet begin to be supplemented? Answering this question requires analysis of infant nutrient requirements, the maximum amount of a specific infant food available, and its nutrient density. Much of the literature on this subject has concentrated on the ability of breast milk to sustain infant growth, primarily because the quantity of breast milk a mother can produce is thought to be biologically limited, while providing other foods is not.

A number of studies on breast milk output have been conducted in high- and low-income countries; Jelliffe and Jelliffe (1978b) and Packard (1982) summarize many of them. A new publication unavailable during the preparation of this book provides additional information on the quantity and quality of breast milk (WHO, 1985). In well-nourished Swedish women breast milk production rose from approximately 550 ml per day in the first two weeks to 750−800 ml by the sixth month, and was higher for mothers of male infants. Women in low-income countries seem to have lower outputs, ranging from 500 to 700 ml in the first six months.

Figures V-1 and V-2 compare average breast milk output of well-nourished women to the amount needed to meet infant energy and protein requirements as determined by several authors. The requirements assume growth along

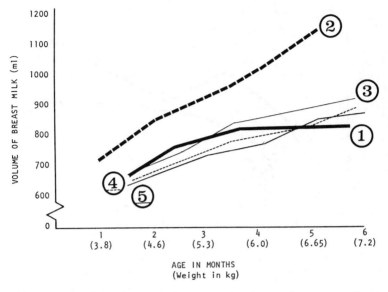

KEY

1 = average breast milk output as reported by Waterlow & Thomson, 1979
Energy requirements according to various calculations:
2 = Passmore et al., 1974
3 = Waterlow & Thomson, 1979
4 = Waterlow & Thomson, revised (see text)
5 = Whitehead & Paul, 1981

FIGURE V-1   Daily volume of breast milk needed to meet infant energy requirements compared with average volume of milk produced by well-nourished women.

the 25th percentile of the NAS standards, and a breast milk composition
of 70 kcal and 1.2 gm protein/100 ml.

By Waterlow and Thomson's calculations (1979), the energy requirements
of an infant growing at the 25th percentile at about age three months would
not be met by the average breast milk output of a well-nourished woman.
However, growth along the fifth percentile could be sustained until at least
the sixth month and growth along the tenth percentile until the fifth month.
The WHO energy requirements would not be met during the first month.
Such analyses are highly sensitive to changes in underlying assumptions.
Calculations of breast milk volume necessary to meet energy requirements
have been made using Fomon's (1967) data on the composition of infant
weight gain. This slight change in requirements pushes back the age at

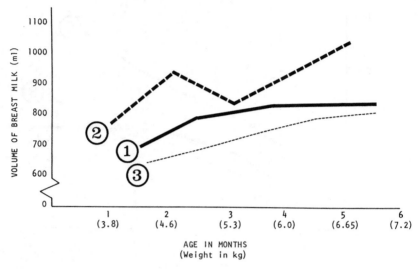

1 = average breast milk output as reported by Waterlow & Thomson, 1979
2 = protein requirements according to WHO calculations by Passmore et al., 1974
3 = protein requirements according to calculations by Waterlow & Thomson, 1979

FIGURE V-2   Daily volume of breast milk needed to meet infant protein requirements compared with average volume of milk produced by well-nourished women.

which the volume of breast milk becomes inadequate to five to six months. With the Whitehead and Paul (1981) calculations of energy requirements, the age at which breast milk is likely to become inadequate is five months. Exclusive breast-feeding at the lower average breast milk outputs reported for women in low-income countries would be inadequate to meet energy needs at considerably earlier ages. See WHO, 1985.

See figure V-2 for analysis of the ability of breast milk to meet infant protein needs. Waterlow and Thomson's calculations reveal that, unlike energy, infant protein requirements can be met by the average volume of breast milk produced by well-nourished women through at least the first six months. However, even a one-month-old infant would not be able to meet the WHO protein recommendation on breast milk alone. A major difference in the results of these analyses is because the WHO protein recommendation includes a margin of safety while Waterlow and Thomson's calculation and the data on breast milk output are based on mean values.

It is therefore more appropriate to compare Waterlow and Thomson's figures with those on breast milk output. If women in low-income countries produce lower volumes of breast milk, exclusive breast-feeding may be inadequate to meet an infant's protein needs at an earlier age.

The underlying assumptions and calculations in analyses of this type are, at present, too imprecise to allow firm conclusions as to an average time when exclusive breast-feeding will be inadequate to meet infant needs for energy and protein. Waterlow *et al.* (1981) conclude there is general agreement that (1) exclusive breast-feeding is usually adequate for the first two months of life; (2) under favorable conditions (a well-nourished, motivated mother, with a high level of support), exclusive breast-feeding can be adequate for up to four to six months; and (3) it will usually be inadequate after six months. There is disagreement whether exclusive breast-feeding can meet infant nutrient needs from two to six months under the less than favorable conditions existing in many low-income countries.

While the amount of breast milk available to an infant may be limited by biological factors such as maternal nutritional status, economic and social factors may limit the quantity of nutrients available to a nonbreast-fed infant. Because of the wide variety of foods used and the lack of information on the quantities fed to infants in low-income countries, it is difficult to determine when and under what conditions each combination of other foods becomes inadequate as a sole source of infant nourishment. Theoretically, commercial infant formula, properly prepared and given in sufficient quantities, should be adequate for six months or longer. Whether these conditions are, or can be, met in low-income countries, given current living conditions, has not been adequately studied. Foods other than infant formula are unlikely to be completely adequate, especially for young infants, particularly cereal-based gruels, which may lack or be low in several nutrients and have a low energy density.

Predicting the consequences of inadequate energy and protein intakes for infants is difficult. Maintenance needs generally cannot change significantly in response to lower intakes. Therefore, energy shortages must be met by reduced physical activity or growth. Because of scarce information on the activity levels of infants, it is not clear how much of an energy deficit can be met by decreasing physical activity. With anything other than mild energy insufficiency, growth will be affected.

Experimental evidence from animal research indicates a higher vulnerability to growth insult with deficient nutrient intakes in young animals (McCance and Widdowson, 1962). Work with young rats showed that this growth insult was irreversible even with adequate feeding later. The high growth rate peculiar to infancy has been used as a basis for speculating that nutrient deficiencies during this period may be of greater significance to overall growth than later deficiencies.

Composition of Infant Foods

Infant foods differ not only in the amounts necessary to meet gross nutrient needs, but also in such aspects as the balance of amino acids and types of fatty acids present that may also influence growth.

Milk composition varies among species (Arman, 1979). Extensive reviews on the subject are available (Blanc, 1981; György, 1971; Jelliffe and Jelliffe, 1971; Jenness, 1974, 1979; Nichols and Nichols, 1979; and Packard, 1982). Infants are fed a variety of milks (cow, human, reindeer, goat, buffalo) and other foods depending on a multitude of sociocultural factors. The nutrient quality of milks differs. It is assumed that each species produces milk to meet the needs of its offspring for nutritional status and growth. How well is the nutrient composition of these milks suited to human needs? In this section we discuss the milks most commonly used (human milk, undiluted cow's milk, and milk-based formula) and biochemical differences in gross nutrient composition, amino-acid content, fatty-acids, vitamins, and minerals as they may affect metabolism, nutritional status, and growth.

A variety of milk-based formulas are available in low- and high-income countries. See table V-4 for a brief description of these formulas; detailed reviews are readily available (Fomon, 1974; WHO, 1985).

Protein

Cow's milk contains three times more protein than human milk, mainly in the form of casein (see table V-5). Formula foods for routine feeding of normal infants (e.g., Enfamil) resemble human milk in total protein content. Since formula manufacturers try to simulate human milk within technological and financial constraints, whey is often combined with nonfat cow's milk to achieve a casein:whey ratio resembling human milk, producing formulas often referred to as "humanized" (e.g., SMA). The quality of casein in cow's and human milk differs. Human milk contains chiefly beta-casein; cow's milk has alpha-2 casein. When casein is precipitated in the stomach, cow's milk forms a tough, rubbery curd; human milk forms a soft, flocculent curd. This difference in curd quality may have two effects:

TABLE V-4

Commercial formulas marketed in Europe and the United States by components

Formula	Manufacturer	Components		
		Protein	Fat	Carbohydrate
EUROPE				
Golden Ostermilk	Glaxo			
Ostermilk Two	Glaxo	Cow milk	Butterfat	None
Utilac 26	Glaxo			
Babymilk 2	Cow & Gate			
Perlargon	Nestlé			
Nido 1ᵉʳ Age	Nestlé	Cow milk	Butterfat	Varies
Milumil	Milupa			
Nidina	Nestlé			
Nektarmil	Milupa		Butterfat	
Tillagg	Findus Semper		&/or	
Lemiel 1	Glaxo	Cow milk	vegetable	Varies
Bebiron	Nutricia		oil	
Multival	Von Heyden			
Trufood	Cow & Gate			
NAN	Nestlé			
Baby Semp	Semper		Vegetable	
Aptamil	Milupa	Cow milk	oil &/or	Varies
Almiron M2	Nutricia	whey	butterfat	
Humana 1	Human			
Pomila	Maizina			
UNITED STATES				Lactose or
Enfamil	Mead Johnson.	Nonfat	Vegetable	corn syrup
Similac	Ross	cow milk	oil	solids
SMA	Wyeth	Demineral-ized whey & nonfat cow milk	Vegetable oil, oleo oil	Lactose

Sources: Adapted from Fomon, 1974 (pp. 378–379); United Kingdom, 1980.

TABLE V-5

Composition of human milk, cow's milk, and milk-based formula

| Nutrient | Human Milk | | | | Cow's Milk | Milk-Based Formula | | |
| | Colostrum | 4–6 | 7–11 | 12–20 | | FDA Minimum (1971)[a] 0–12 mos | AAPCNR (1976)[a] | Formula (e.g., Enfamil) |
		Infant Age in Months						
Water				87.6 g/dl	87.6 g/dl			
Energy	67 kcal/dl			71 kcal/dl	69 kcal/dl	67 kcal/dl	67 kcal/dl	68 kcal/dl
Total Solids				12.9 g/dl	12.8 g/dl			
Protein	10 g/dl	1.26 g/dl	1.24 g/dl	1.1 g/dl	3.5 g/dl	1.8 g	1.8–4.5 g	1.5–1.6 g/dl
Casein				40% of TP	82% of TP			
Whey Protein	1.6 g/dl			60% of TP	18% of TP			
Beta Lactoglobulin				0	.3 g/dl			
Alpha Lactalbumin	1.1 g/dl			263 mg/dl	.3–.4 g/dl			
Lactoferrin	1.4 g/dl			168 mg/dl	trace			
Lysozyme				42 mg/dl	trace			
Serum/ Albumin				52 mg/dl	40 mg/dl			
IgA				142 mg/dl				
Amino Acids Essential				.4 g/dl	1.6 g/dl			
Leucine				100 mg/dl	350 mg/dl			150 mg/dl
Lysine				73 mg/dl	277 mg/dl			124 mg/dl
Valine				70 mg/dl	245 mg/dl			96 mg/dl
Isoleucine				68 mg/dl	228 mg/dl			80 mg/dl
Threonine				50 mg/dl	164 mg/dl			69 mg/dl
Phenylalanine				48 mg/dl	172 mg/dl			73 mg/dl
Methionine				25 mg/dl	88 mg/dl			39 mg/dl
Histidine				22 mg/dl	95 mg/dl			45 mg/dl
Tryptophan				18 mg/dl	49 mg/dl			26 mg/dl

TABLE V-5 (continued)

Nutrient	Human Milk					Milk-Based Formula		
	Infant Age in Months				Cow's Milk	FDA Minimum (1971)[a] 0–12 mos	AAPCNR (1976)[a]	Formula (e.g., Enfamil)
	Colostrum	4–6	7–11	12–20				
Amino Acids								
Nonessential								
Glutamic acid				230 mg/dl	680 mg/dl			
Aspartic acid				116 mg/dl	166 mg/dl			
Proline				80 mg/dl	250 mg/dl			
Serine				69 mg/dl	160 mg/dl			
Tyrosine				61 mg/dl	179 mg/dl			
Arginine				45 mg/dl	129 mg/dl			60 mg/dl
Alanine				35 mg/dl	75 mg/dl			
Cystine				24 mg/dl	13 mg/dl			13 mg/dl
Fat	2.9 g/dl	4.41 g/dl	3.45 g/dl	4–4.8 g/dl	3.7 g/dl	1.7 g	3.3–6.0 g	3.7–3.8 g/dl
Fatty Acids								
Essential (% saturated)								
Shorter than C12				2%	9%			3%
C12 & longer					53%			28%
(% poly-unsaturated)				9%	4%			49%
Triglyceride (% of total fatty acids)								
12:0 Lauric				1.5%	2.7%			
14:0 Myristic				5.2%	11.0%			
16:0 Palmitic				25.6%	29.9%			

TABLE V-5 (continued)

Nutrient	Human Milk				Cow's Milk	Milk-Based Formula		
	Colostrum	Infant Age in Months				FDA Minimum (1971)[a] 0–12 mos	AAPCNR (1976)[a]	Formula (e.g., Enfamil)
		4–6	7–11	12–20				
Triglyceride (% of total fatty acids)								
16:1 Palmitoleic				2.7%	3.1			
18:0 Stearic				8.4%	12.9			
18:1 Oleic				35.6%	29.1			
18:2 n-6 Linoleic				8.7%	2.1			
18:3 n-3 Linolenic				3.4%	1.9			
C20 & C22 PUFA				6.60%	1.20			
Phospholipids (% of total phospholipids)								
Phosphatidyl Ethanolamine				36.6%	22.3			
Phosphatidyl Choline				29.7%	33.6			
Sphingomyelin				26.2%	35.3			
Phosphatidyl Inositol				4.6%	2.0			
Lysolecithin				1.9%	1.0			
Phosphatidyl Serine				1.0%	2.3			
Cerebrosides				—	1.8			
Cholestrol	27 mg/dl			20 mg/dl	14 mg/dl			27 mg/dl

TABLE V-5 (continued)

Nutrient	Human Milk					Milk-Based Formula		
	Colostrum	Infant Age in Months			Cow's Milk	FDA Minimum (1971)[a] 0–12 mos	AAPCNR (1976)[a]	Formula (e.g., Enfamil)
		4–6	7–11	12–20				
Vitamins								
A	151 µg/dl			57 µg/dl; 190 µg/dl	45.30 µg/dl; 103 IU/dl	250 IU	250–270 IU	51–79.5 µg/dl; 169 IU/dl
D	1.78 µg/dl			1.0 µg/dl; 2.2 IU/dl	1.05 µg/dl; 3.4 IU/dl	40 IU	40–100 IU	1–1.05 µg/dl; 42 IU/dl
E	1.5 mg/dl			.9 IU/dl	.1 IU/dl	.3 IU	.3 IU	.9–1.5 IU/dl
K							4 µg	
Thiamin	1.9 µg/dl			3.4 µg/dl	17 µg/dl	25 µg	40 µg	52–70 µg/dl
Riboflavin	30 µg/dl			16 µg/dl	44 µg/dl	60 µg	60 µg	63–106 µg/dl
Niacin	75 µg/dl			36 µg/dl; 1.50 mg/dl	175 µg/dl; .90 mg/dl			.70–1 mg/dl
B_6	.05 µg/dl			10 µg/dl	66 µg/dl	35 µg	35 µg	40–42 µg/dl
B_{12}				.03 µg/dl	.4 µg/dl	.15 µg	.15 µg	.1–.2 µg/dl
Folacin	.05 µg/dl			2.80 µg/dl	2 µg/dl	4 µg	4 µg	5–10 µg/dl
C	5.9 mg/dl			4.30 mg/dl	.82 mg/dl	7.8 mg	8 mg	5.2–5.8 mg/dl
Pantothenic acid	183 µl/dl			190 µg/dl		300 µg	300 µg	
Minerals								
Calcium	39 mg/dl	24.8 mg/dl	23.6 mg/dl	20–33 mg/dl	125 mg/dl	50 mg	50 mg	45–58 mg/dl
Phosphorus	14 mg/dl			15 mg/dl	96 mg/dl	25 mg	25 mg	33–46 mg/dl
Magnesium	4 mg/dl	3.33 mg/dl	3.19 mg/dl	3–4 mg/dl	12 mg/dl	6 mg	6 mg	3.9–5.3 mg/dl
Iron	70 µg/dl	21 µl/dl	18 µg/dl	20–24 µg/dl	.10 mg/dl	1 mg	.15 mg	trace–1.30 mg/d
Zinc		.079 mg/dl	.042 mg/dl	.033–.16 mg/dl	.38 mg/dl	—	.5 mg	.36–.50 mg/dl
Copper	.04 µg/dl	.023 mg/dl	.017 mg/dl	.02 mg/dl	.06 mg/dl	.06 mg	.06 mg	.04–.07 mg/dl

TABLE V-5 (continued)

Nutrient	Human Milk				Cow's Milk	Milk-Based Formula		
	Infant Age in Months					FDA Minimum (1971)[a] 0–12 mos	AAPCNR (1976)[a]	Formula (e.g., Enfamil)
	Colostrum	4–6	7–11	12–20				
Minerals								
Chloride	85 mg/dl			38.5 mg/dl			53 mg/dl	53 mg/dl
Potassium	74 mg/dl	44.3 mg/dl	38.9 mg/dl	40–55 mg/dl			70 mg/dl	70 mg/dl
Sodium	48 mg/dl	11.3 mg/dl	84 mg/dl	10–15 mg/dl			28 mg/dl	38 mg/dl
Carbohydrate								
Lactose	5.3 g/dl	7.71 g/dl	7.57 g/dl	7.23 g/dl	4.9 g/dl			5.3 g/dl

Sources: AAP, 1976; Blanc, 1981; Drew et al., 1984; Jelliffe & Jelliffe, 1978a; Jenness, 1979; Lakdawala & Widdowson, 1977; Mead Johnson, 1977; Nayman et al., 1979; Watson et al., 1980.

[a]Per 100 kcal unless otherwise specified.

Notes: AAPCNR = American Academy of Pediatrics Committee on Nutrition Recommendations; FDA = Food and Drug Administration; TP = total protein; PUFA = polyunsaturated fatty acids

(1) gastrointestinal transit time (Fomon, 1974) may be faster in infants fed cow's milk or formula, altering (decreasing) absorption of nutrients, or providing a more inconsistent energy supply, and (2) the tougher curd may be more difficult to digest. Human milk is also rich in whey proteins and differs from cow's milk in lacking beta-lactoglobulin. The higher protein content of certain milks may be manifested as increases in urea levels. Davies and Saunders (1973) and Dale et al. (1975) found nonbreast-fed infants had high mean blood urea levels compared to breast-fed infants, with infants fed unmodified cow's milk formula (high protein content) having higher levels than those fed humanized milk formula. The increases observed have not been shown to be harmful, although their significance requires clinical evaluation.

Rassin et al. (1978) found quantitative and qualitative differences in essential amino-acid content of milks. Cow's milk contains higher levels than human milk, while milk-based formulas (e.g., Enfamil) have levels only slightly higher than human milk.

Protein quality may also differ. The lower level of cystine in cow's milk and milk-based formula is significant for premature infants who lack the enzyme cystothionase which converts methionine to cystine. Cystine may be essential for premature and very young infants (Sturman et al., 1970). Premature infants are also limited in their ability to metabolize tyrosine and phenylalanine. Tyrosine is much higher in cow's milk; phenylalanine is highest in cow's milk, lowest in human milk, with levels in formula lying in between (Table V-5). Cow's milk may therefore burden premature and perhaps term infants with quantities of these amino acids they cannot handle. Effects may include aminoacidemia (Mamunes et al., 1976), leading to neuropathological alterations. It has also been hypothesized that the human infant cannot synthesize the amino acid taurine, usually absent in formulas although no obvious clinical signs have been observed in formula-fed infants. Effects of this absence are unknown although it may alter brain development (Sturman et al., 1977a, b).

Finally, human milk contains a variety of nucleotides, whereas cow's milk contains primarily orotic acid. Polyamines are also present in higher amounts in human milk than in cow's milk. The high levels of both these components in human milk may enhance synthesis of protein, an essential phenomenon for growth (Sanguansermsri et al., 1974) and brain development.

Fat

Fat provides the bulk of calories in all milks. Fat quality and quantity differ in different kinds of milk. Formula may contain butterfat, vegetable oils (soy, coconut, or both), or a combination of the two. The amounts of saturated and polyunsaturated fat may thus also vary. Table V-5 includes further details on fats and fatty acids. An infant suckling at the breast receives varying quantities of fat depending on time of day and feeding duration. The fat content of human milk is usually high in the morning, plateauing at midday. Hindmilk, the last milk taken during a feeding, is three times higher in fat content than foremilk (Hall, 1979). Hall (1975) has suggested that the change in fat content during a breast-feeding signals the infant to stop feeding and thereby acts as an appetite control mechanism. A bottle-fed infant is deprived of this effect.

Although effects of these fat differences on an infant's nutritional status and metabolism require further study, a few have been hypothesized to be expected. Fomon (1974) and others have observed differences in fat excretion depending on type of milk consumed, thought to have little effect on the infant's health. Since the amount of polyunsaturated fatty acids (PUFA) varies with the type of milk ingested, requirements for vitamin E may be altered; excessive PUFA results in excessive tissue peroxidation. This is of concern with infants fed formulas extremely high in PUFA and low in vitamin E, and in premature infants. Variation in fatty-acid content may alter body fat composition. A great deal more research is necessary before the consequences of this difference, possibly related to obesity and degenerative diseases in adulthood, are understood. Widdowson *et al.* (1975) and others indicate that body fat composition varies with fat type in a formula.

Reiser and Sidelman (1972) have hypothesized that cholesterol levels in milk in early life may help establish a mechanism for maintaining low serum cholesterol levels in adulthood. Human milk is higher in cholesterol than cow's milk or formula. Reiser and Sidelman worked with rats; we cannot be sure that this mechanism functions in human infants. Ginsburg and Zetterström (1980) measured the increase in lipid levels from cord blood to serum at three to six months and found significantly greater increases in total cholesterol and high-density lipid cholesterol among exclusively breast-fed infants compared to other babies. Freidman and Goldberg (1975) and Patricia A. Hodgson *et al.* (1976) provided evidence of no protection against high serum cholesterol levels *later in life* as a consequence of receiving increased levels of cholesterol during infancy. Furthermore, maternal diet influences human milk cholesterol levels, thereby leading to a wide variation in cholesterol levels (Jensen *et al.*, 1978; Picciano *et al.*, 1978), further repudiating this hypothesis.

Presence of inadequate amounts of essential fatty acids such as linoleic acid in cow's milk formulas is of concern, although it is believed that the minimal requirements for this nutrient have been overestimated (Cuthbertson, 1976; Naismith *et al.*, 1978). Sanders and Naismith (1979) detected lower levels of long-chain polyunsaturated derivatives of linoleic and linolenic acids in the erythrocyte lipids of infants fed cow's milk formulas compared to breast-fed infants, although essential fatty acid deficiency was not noted. Therefore, it seems that infants fed formulas are at no immediate risk of fatty acid deficiency.

Human milk has been shown to have higher levels of long-chain polyene acids such as arachidonic acid, implicated in the development of the brain and nervous system (Sinclair and Crawford, 1972). The importance of elevated levels of arachidonic acids in human milk is controversial. Olegard and Svennerholm (1971, as cited in Sanders and Naismith, 1979) found no significant differences in the proportion of arachidonic acid in plasma and erythrocyte phosphoglycerides of three-month old infants fed either breast milk or a skimmed milk formula containing vegetable fat. (Skimmed milk formulas and vegetable fat are extremely low in arachidonic acid.)

Although the high lipase levels in human milk are often referred to as beneficial in making fatty acids more available (György, 1971), Jensen and colleagues (1978) present evidence suggesting this is unlikely.

Finally, human milk has higher levels of palmitic acid in the 2 position whereas cow's milk contains palmitic acid in the 1 and 3 positions. Jelliffe and Jelliffe (1978a) suggest that palmitic acid in the 2 position is more easily absorbed. Formula contains little palmitic acid. The relevance of absorbance of formula fat to the above information remains unclear. The influence of fat on calcium absorption is important since palmitic acid in the 1 and 3 positions may be precipitated by calcium in the intestine, forming calcium-palmitate soap, thereby increasing the loss of calcium and fat.

Carbohydrate

Lactose is the main carbohydrate component in most milks used for normal infants. More recently corn syrup solids have been substituted in infant formulas. Numerous researchers have felt that lactose may enhance calcium absorption and thereby prevent rickets (Lengemann, 1959). According to Allen (1982:794), "These data suggest that lactose intolerance has a negligible effect on calcium absorption, although this needs to be confirmed in long-term balance study."

Minerals

Most mineral levels in cow's milk are approximately three times higher than in the same amount of human milk (table V-5) contributing to an estimated renal solute load of 23mOsm/dl for infants fed whole cow's milk, as compared to 7.5mOsm/dl for infants fed human milk, and 11mOsm/dl for infants fed formula (Mead Johnson, 1977). Metabolic and physiologic problems from the high osmolar quality of some milks may be manifested as increased water loss, dehydration, fever, diarrhea, vomiting, and possible brain damage (Rosenbloom and Sills, 1975). High levels of electrolytes have also been detected in the vitreous humor of dead infants (Emery *et al.*, 1974), indicating that high solute feeding and water deficiency may have been involved in the deaths. During illnesses such as gastroenteritis and dehydration, the adequacy of minerals in human milk is questionable (Kingston, 1975).

The iron content of human and cow's milk is low, although iron in human milk is much better absorbed than either iron from cow's milk or nonfortified formulas (Jelliffe and Jelliffe, 1978a, b; McMillan *et al.*, 1976). Most formulas may be purchased with or without added iron. Iron concentration in human milk is affected by maternal diet and period of lactation. Iron concentration decreases during the course of lactation (from about .52 to .3mg/l) (Anaokar and Garry, 1981; Siimes *et al.*, 1971). Surprisingly, this superior bioavailability of iron from human milk is compromised by presence in the diet of other foods (Oski and Landaw, 1980:459).

For approximately the first four months of life, infants draw on liver stores of iron after which they become more dependent on diet to meet iron requirements. Therefore, for the first four months, a wholly breast-fed infant is not expected to be deficient in iron, provided (1) prenatally acquired iron stores are adequate (depending in turn on maternal nutritional status during pregnancy), and (2) no unusual blood loss occurs to increase iron requirements (Wilson *et al.*, 1964). Iron deficiency does not occur with formulas diluted as recommended. Breast-fed infants have been found to have serum iron levels as high as infants fed iron-fortified formulas and higher than those of infants fed nonfortified formulas (Picciano and Deering, 1980). Much controversy on the adequacy of human milk iron continues and the necessity for supplementation is still debated (Bullen *et al.*, 1978; Garry *et al.*, 1981; McMillan *et al.*, 1976; Owen *et al.*, 1981; Saarinen,

1978). Fomon and Strauss (1978) believe supplementation is nutritionally necessary, yet it may alter the bacteriostatic effect of lactoferrin among breast-fed infants.

Although calcium in human milk is lower than in cow's milk or formulas, it is better absorbed (Jelliffe and Jelliffe, 1978a). Decreased absorption of calcium from cow's milk may be attributed to fat quality, high phosphate content, or lactose content.

The bioavailability of zinc in human milk appears to be higher than in cow's milk or formulas which may in turn affect other metabolic aspects because of zinc deficiencies (Casey et al., 1981; Duncan and Hurley, 1978; Goodhart and Shils, 1980; Hambidge et al., 1979; Piletz and Ganschow, 1979; Sändström, 1983).

Vitamins

Human milk contains higher levels of vitamins A, C, and E than cow's milk. Table V-5 includes levels in milk-based formulas. Amounts of vitamin E are proportionate to amounts of PUFAs present; this is important in preventing excessive peroxidation precipitated by the presence of high levels of PUFAs. Although most formulas are high in PUFAs, manufacturers usually make the required adjustments.

Vitamin K levels are lower in human milk. The newborn obtains vitamin K from fetal liver stores until intestinal organisms capable of synthesizing it are established. If vitamin K levels decrease to unusually low levels in the newborn, the threat of hemorrhagic diseases is of concern. Vitamin K adequacy in human milk is a matter of controversy.

The quantity of vitamin D in milks is similar (see table V-5). Scientists have debated its adequacy in human milk (Reeve et al., 1982). Many feel supplements are essential. Cases have been reported of black, breast-fed infants who developed vitamin D deficiency rickets (Bachrach et al., 1979; Edidin et al., 1980). The numbers of these cases do not appear sufficient to conclude that breast-fed infants are at risk of developing rickets; the issue is worthy of further exploration using comparison groups. Under normal conditions, in which the mother ingests adequate amounts of vitamin D and receives vitamin D through exposure to sunlight, human milk is expected to provide sufficient amounts of vitamin D for normal growth and development.

Craft et al. (1971), Ford et al. (1975), and Gullberg (1974) show the significance of low levels of vitamin B_{12} and increased levels of unsaturated B_{12}-binding protein in human milk. Human milk contains that protein which makes the vitamin, unavailable to intestinal organisms that depend on these vitamins for survival. The B_{12}-binding protein may increase the bioavailability of the vitamin to the infant, decreasing its availability to bacteria dependent on it, thereby changing intestinal flora in the gut.

Pollutants

Human milk may also contain pollutants ingested by the lactating woman. These are usually lipid-soluble, resistant to physical degradation or metabolism, widely distributed in the environment, and slowly excreted or not at all (Rogan *et al.*, 1980). Polychlorinate biphenyls (PCBs) and dichlorodiphenyl trichloroethane (DDT) are two chemicals of well-known concern since higher than safe levels have been detected in human milk (Arena, 1980; Poland and Cohen, 1980; Rogan *et al.*, 1980; Wickizer and Brilliant, 1981). Maternal consumption of drugs of various kinds (alcohol, heroin, senna, thiouracil) and hormones such as oral contraceptives are reflected in milk quality (Arena, 1980; Koldovsky, 1980). The significance of their presence in human milk is unknown. Since many of these substances are known to be detrimental to adults, they could also be harmful to infants. Effects at the same dose may be more pronounced in the infant because of its smaller body mass.

Factors Affecting Quality of Human Milk

Variation in nutrient composition of human milk directly affects infant nutritional status and metabolism. Studies by Lindblad and Rahimtoola (1974) on milk of poorly nourished women in Pakistan indicated an amino-acid content similar to that of well-nourished women, although methionine and lysine levels were lower.

Quality of dietary fat and quantity of carbohydrate ingested by the mother may influence fatty-acid patterns in milk (Aitchison *et al.*, 1977; Read *et al.*, 1965). Mothers consuming diets high in polyunsaturated fatty acids show increased levels of these acids in their milk (Kramer *et al.*, 1965; Sanders *et al.*, 1984), with a consequent change in the polyunsaturated:saturated fatty acid ratio along with changes in cholesterol levels (Potter and Nestel, 1976). Among poorly nourished women, milk fat levels are reduced, so energy levels may be lower than in the milk of well-nourished women (Jelliffe and Jelliffe, 1978b).

The level of water-soluble vitamins in milk is affected by their amounts in the mother's diet (Jathar *et al.*, 1970; Rajalakshmi *et al.*, 1974; Simpson and Chow, 1956). Vitamin A levels in human milk also seem to reflect the quality of pregnancy and postnatal diet and maternal nutritional status. Prenatal and postnatal vitamin A supplementation of women in Central America was followed by a rise in vitamin A levels in breast milk (Arroyave *et al.*, 1974). Dewey and colleagues (1984) studied nutrient levels in human milk in California (table V-5). Concentrations of zinc, copper, and potassium decreased progressively over time (from 4 to 20 months); protein, iron, and sodium declined during the first 6 months and showed no further decline. In addition, weaning was associated with a change in nutrient concentration and amount of milk consumed daily. If milk volume fell below 300ml/day, the concentration of protein and sodium increased while lactose, calcium, and zinc decreased.

Other factors affecting quality of human milk are the stage of nursing and daily variation. Similar research has been done using vitamin C supplements (Bates *et al.*, 1983). A dietary supplement equivalent to 700 kcal given to women in a West African village for 12 months resulted in a slight increase in body weight and subcutaneous fat stores but not in breast milk volume or fat content (Coward *et al.*, 1984; Prentice *et al.*, 1980). During periods of starvation, the significant metabolic consequences may in turn affect nutrient quality of milk (Prentice *et al.*, 1983b). Use of oral contraceptives has also been implicated in alterations observed in the nutrient composition of human milk, although there is much controversy on this subject (McCann *et al.*, 1981).

Conclusions

From the information presented above, it appears possible that exclusive breast-feeding by women in low-income countries may not meet the energy needs of some infants after about three or four months. Exclusive breast-feeding appears to meet protein needs for a longer period of time, until about six months, although with low energy intakes, protein may be diverted from tissue building to catabolization for energy. Infant formula is likely to meet infant nutrient needs for a longer period if prepared properly and in adequate supply. Little is also known about the ability of other foods to meet infant nutrient needs. While breast-feeding may not meet nutrient needs beyond a certain age, it is not known whether under conditions in low-income countries, other foods are equally able to meet infant requirements. Research on this issue is needed.

Energy deficits in infancy lead to a lower growth rate, or, if severe, to cessation of growth. Because of the rapid growth in early infancy, energy deficits at that time may be more detrimental than deficiencies later in life. The specific details of this relationship are not clear. Thus, if a particular feeding method becomes nutritionally inadequate at three rather than six months, the effects on growth may be proportionately greater.

Although infant formulas are designed to resemble the composition of human milk, many differences still exist. The composition of other animal milks differ even more from human milk. Although the differences are well documented, consequences for the infant have not been adequately studied. There is some information on the potential effect of the composition of different foods on biochemical indicators of nutritional status, such as electrolyte levels and iron status, or on the development of specific organs, such as the brain and central nervous system, but there is little biological evidence on how differences in composition may affect growth. Differences in the type of protein may affect growth. The protein from human milk is more completely digested and absorbed and has a more appropriate balance of amino acids. The type of fat found in human milk may favor better growth through the better digestion and absorption of fatty acids themselves and by the favorable effect of fats on calcium absorption. Improved calcium absorption also occurs in the presence of lactose, which is higher in human milk than in infant formula. Calcium absorption affects bone growth which, in turn, affects height. The high osmolarity of cow's milk may result in dehydration, fever, and diarrhea which collectively hinder growth.

Although differences in milk composition may affect infant growth, current knowledge suggests the effects will be minor when compared with those of differences in the gross quantity of nutrients available through different feeding methods. If milk composition does affect growth, it is likely to be stronger if human milk is compared to other animal milks than to properly prepared infant formula. See WHO, 1985.

Significance

The long-term consequences of nutritionally induced growth retardation in infancy are not yet clear. Recovery from an episode of nutrient deficit resulting in growth retardation appears possible. Prader *et al.* (1963) showed that catch-up growth is possible even when nutritional deficits occur early in infancy and persist over several years. Prader and colleagues demonstrated that growth was accelerated in children undergoing rehabilitation and in most cases by adolescence they attained normal growth as measured anthropometrically. Some studies examining this phenomenon among formerly malnourished infants have found that catch-up growth occurred; in others it did not (Garrow and Pike, 1967; Graham and Adrianzen, 1972). The pediatric literature states that catch-up growth is possible if the growth insult occurs before puberty, but it also depends on the timing, length, and severity of the insult (Barr, 1972). Where there is an environmental (sociofamilial) component or the nutritional deficit is secondary to a chronic illness, catch-up growth is not expected. Few data specify or document the mechanism by which catch-up growth operates on its determinants. Until these questions are addressed it is not possible to predict whether and under what conditions a nutritional insult in infancy will result in permanent growth retardation.

EPIDEMIOLOGICAL EVIDENCE

Methodological Issues

That infant feeding may independently affect either morbidity and death, or nutritional status and growth, are analogous types of hypotheses presenting similar methodologic problems. Many of these issues have been discussed in chapter 4. Issues emphasized here are relevant to relationships among infant feeding, nutritional status, and growth.

Measurement and choice of the outcome variable

Growth is the most commonly measured indicator of nutritional status. Compared to biochemical measurements, growth measurements are inexpensive, noninvasive, and accessible. Possible measurements include length (height), weight, head circumference, and skinfold thicknesses. These measures may be expressed as weight/height, weight/height^2, height/$\sqrt[3]{weight}$, mean percentage of expected weight for age, weight gain since birth, status compared with a given percentile of a given set of standards, median growth velocity, median growth velocity/unit of body size, weight gain velocity, and so on. Because weight is easier to measure than height in the first year, many studies collect only weight data during this period.

Weight can be lost, but not height, and weight loss or gain can be immediately responsive to changes in nutritional status. Both characteristics make weight a sensitive indicator of infant nutritional status. The ages, frequencies, and choice of measurements, and their expression as discrete or continuous variables all have implications for study design and statistical analysis, with great variability in choice and expression of the outcome variable.

Biochemical measurements are less suited for field studies. They depend on medical facilities and are expensive and invasive. The advantage of measuring biochemical characteristics is that they may be more specifically related to nutrient intake than growth. Biochemical parameters studied in connection with infant-feeding practices include hemoglobin or hematocrit, serum iron, plasma and red blood cell folate, percentage saturation of transferrin, cholesterol and lipid levels, serum and urine electrolyte levels, and bilirubin levels.

While there is a wide variety of characteristics to measure, a problem arises in choosing appropriate standards with which to compare the observed nutritional and growth measurements. This is less of a problem in studying mortality and morbidity because the outcomes are placed along a continuum from negative (death and high morbidity levels) to positive (no death or illness). The positive outcomes of measuring nutritional status and growth are generally optima in the center of a scale, with outcomes at either end of the scale considered negative. For example, when evaluating weight gain, insufficient and excessive rates are considered negative outcomes. Presently, some breast-feeding advocates (Jelliffe and Jelliffe, 1978a) propose a two-sided hypothesis: that breast-fed infants are less likely to be obese or to be undernourished—thus, their growth is closest to an optimal level. Until this optimal level is clearly defined, it will be difficult to test this two-sided hypothesis.

Classification of the exposure variable: Infant feeding

When testing hypotheses related to infant feeding, nutritional status, and growth, it is essential to quantify the infant's intake of various foods and estimate the amount of nutrients ingested. Interpretations of studies to date implicitly assume that intakes of diets compared are similar, and observed differences in growth may be attributable to diet quality. No published epidemiological study has measured volume and type of food ingested and then compared growth of infants fed different diets. Theoretically it would be interesting to compare the growth of infants fed similar amounts of different diets such as breast milk or formula. In practice it is quite difficult to measure dietary intake in infants, especially breast-fed babies, and variation in quantity may have to be considered an intrinsic characteristic of the food source being studied. Breast milk supply is variable and affected by many factors discussed below, while formula is liable to improper preparation, overconcentration, or overdilution, affecting the amount of nutrients available to the infant.

Measurement of quantity of food and nutrients ingested by the infant

Direct measurement of the volume and composition of the breast milk the infant ingests would be helpful in evaluating the effect of breast-feeding on infant growth. Methods of comparing relative quantities of breast milk produced and ingested include test weighings of infants before and after feeding, expression of breast milk samples at a preset time each day or before or after a feeding, use of heavy water (^2H_2O), or a nipple shield sampling system. Each method involves considerable cost and the first two methods represent interventions in themselves. Test weighings before and after feedings are simple in theory, needing only immediate access to a scale, but the method has serious problems. Measuring a mother's "performance" may cause anxiety and thus affect breast-feeding success (de Chateau *et al.*, 1977). This procedure interferes with the spontaneous interaction conducive to successful breast-feeding. In societies where breast-feeding is frequent and the infant suckles day and night, test weighings will interfere with the pattern of breast-feeding, and it may be difficult to measure all feedings in a given time period, and the small amounts ingested in each feeding. In several studies (Edozien, 1979; Hennart and Vis, 1980), women were hospitalized for the test period, to allow easier measurement and weighings. Such hospitalization is bound to affect the breast-feeding relationship.

Using pumps to express milk also has several drawbacks. The sample is usually taken at preset times—first thing in the morning or one hour after a feeding (Sosa *et al.*, 1976). These methods allow relative comparisons of breast milk production in a cross-sectional study, but because of the potential effect of the pump on prolactin levels and milk supply, it is not appropriate to take frequent, serial samples by this method.

In the heavy water technique a small amount of ^2H_2O is injected into the infant and its appearance and dilution in the saliva are measured over the course of 11 to 14 days. This technique appears to be accurate (Coward *et al.*, 1979), producing results similar to those obtained by test weighing, although its accuracy on an individual basis has been disputed (Butte *et al.*, 1983). The laboratory tests required make this technique expensive, but Coward and colleagues feel that, aside from financial constraints, this method is feasible in a variety of international settings. Coward *et al.* (1982) have since modified the technique for the situation when the baby is drinking other liquids in addition to breast milk. In this case ^2H_2O is administered to the mother.

In the nipple shield sampling system, a latex nipple shield equipped with a sampling line is placed on the breast and electronically measures the rate of flow (Lucas *et al.*, 1980; Woolridge *et al.*, 1982). This method involves the use of electronic equipment, is probably expensive or unwieldy in a field setting, and may not be acceptable to all mothers or all cultures.

Because of the difficulties in measuring the amount of breast milk produced and ingested, there is need to develop better measurement techniques and to find more easily measured variables which correlate well with quantity. A review of factors affecting breast milk quantity may point the direction for research in this area, although at present there is no one variable that can serve as a proxy for quantity.

Measuring the quantity of other foods the infant ingests is considerably easier than measuring breast milk, although problems do exist. The age of the infant may affect measurements; older infants may obtain food that the mother or other informant is unaware of. When quantities of other foods ingested are measured, their quality should also be sampled, especially in the case of formula feeding where the dilution as well as total volume ingested needs to be determined (Surjono *et al.*, 1980).

Factors affecting the amount of food ingested by the infant

The amount of food available and offered to the infant is affected by economic and cultural factors. Some mothers dilute formula because of economic necessity; some overconcentrate formula because of inadequate education; some overfeed their babies because of certain cultural expectations. Improper dilution of formula is a major problem (Surjono *et al.*, 1980), and only by measuring quantity as well as concentration of formula is it possible to know the amount of nutrients the infant receives.

Studies measuring breast milk production have found 24-hour volumes to vary from 340 to 1200 ml (Worthington-Roberts *et al.*, 1985). Physiological factors may affect breast milk supply, including maternal nutritional status (Gopalan, 1958; Hanafy *et al.*, 1972; Hennart and Vis, 1980; Khin-Maung-Naing *et al.*, 1980; Prentice *et al.*, 1980; Whitehead *et al.*, 1978), stage of lactation (Gopalan, 1958; Hanafy *et al.*, 1972), and narcotic or pharmaceutical use, especially of oral contraceptives (McCann *et al.*, 1981).

Cultural factors may also affect breast milk availability. Brazleton (1977), Simpson-Hebert (1980), and others have noted a great contrast between breast-feeding and mother-infant interaction in traditional non-Western societies and modern, industrialized societies. A constellation of behaviors and practices characterize the former: (1) carrying the infant close to the body in a pack or sling; (2) sleeping with the infant; (3) wearing clothing which allows easy, frequent access to the breast; (4) encouraging frequent suckling for nutritive and nonnutritive purposes, on the slightest sound from the infant, and, after several months, suckling on the infant's initiative; (5) continuing breast-feeding into the second year and beyond (Simpson-Hebert, 1980). Between this pattern and that of modern, industrial societies—virtually the opposite in every respect—are a variety of cultural patterns that determine styles of dress, sleeping, and work; acceptability of breast-feeding in public; and the compatability of breast-feeding with other female roles. Cultural beliefs may also be manifested as attitudes toward infant size, growth, and gratification of infant demands (Ainsworth, 1977). All these cultural mechanisms may affect the infant's access to the breast, and frequency and length of feedings, in turn affecting prolactin levels, milk production, and the amount ingested.

Confounding variables

Variables predicting growth and independently associated with choice of feeding method are potential confounders. These variables probably affect growth by affecting the infant's level of morbidity or the amount of nutrients available to it. The type of health care available to the family may affect the mother's choice of feeding method, and determine the medical care the infant receives when ill. Family economic status may be associated with the mother's feeding choice and simultaneously affect the amount of food available to the infant. Were it possible to control for episodes of morbidity and quantity of food ingested by the infant, there might not be many other confounding variables. If these two variables cannot be measured in a study, then it becomes necessary to control for variables associated with morbidity and quantity of nutrients, and to think carefully about the selection of such potential confounders.

Another variable which may be an important confounder is the infant's initial size, expressed as birth weight and gestational age. Of particular concern are small for gestational age (SGA) infants. Unfortunately, many studies in developing countries do not measure either birth weight or gestational age, and it is not clear how these variables are related to the mother's feeding decisions. They probably predict morbidity and growth patterns, and if associated with feeding decisions, may be confounders in studies which compare two groups of infants fed different diets. Methods for collecting gestational age data in the field exist (e.g., Ballard *et al.*, 1979). Nevertheless, most research or gestational age assessment has been clinic or hospital based (Dubowitz *et al.*, 1970).

Study design issues

Two important design issues when measuring the effect of infant diet on growth are choice of comparison group and longitudinal versus cross-sectional sampling. Studies either compare two groups of infants fed different diets and measure their growth, or they compare growth of one group of infants to that of another used as standards for growth, for example, the NCHS 1979 standards. The first is the more traditional epidemiological approach. Both groups of infants are drawn from the same population, during the same period. The same data are collected uniformly for each group and an effort can be made to assess and control for confounding. Appropriate statistical tests can be conducted. The main disadvantages of this approach are that better growth may not be clearly defined and results may be difficult to compare with other studies. An example of the first problem would be in modern, industrialized settings where there is some dispute whether more growth is better or not. In observing growth differences in two middle-class populations of infants, one breast-fed, one formula-fed, one must still interpret the differences and assign them some meaning.

Comparing the growth of one study group to that of a group of infants now used as standards (from here on described as standard infants) saves expense and allows comparison of results across studies. This method precludes assessing or controlling for confounding, or conducting statistical analyses. Its major drawback is choosing an appropriate standard—a problem receiving much recent attention (Hitchcock *et al.*, 1981; Neumann, 1979; Seward and Serdula, 1984; Whitehead and Paul, 1984). The main points raised are that (1) very small sample sizes were used to construct the infant portions of most currently used growth charts; (2) data were often collected cross-sectionally rather than longitudinally; (3) infant samples were drawn over a long period of time, from as early as 1929, and were fed quite differently from infants of today; (4) infants were probably not breast-fed and their growth patterns may not be an appropriate model for breast-fed infants; (5) the standard infants' growth may not be relevant for SGA infants—a large proportion of babies in developing countries. Using inappropriate standards may result in misclassifying infants as undernourished, and even if the misclassification is the same (nondifferential) in all feeding groups being compared, it may lead to a conservative bias, towards the null hypothesis (Kleinbaum et al., 1982). Inappropriate standards may also lead to incorrect recomendations regarding the best time to introduce other foods to the breast-fed infant, as Whitehead and Paul (1984) illustrate and discuss well.

Whether one compares growth of two groups of infants fed differently or of one infant group to that of a set of growth standards, the researcher has the choice of a cross-sectional or longitudinal design. Cross-sectional designs, where anthropometric measurements are taken from a group of infants at different ages, have disadvantages of not allowing the researcher (1) to assess the temporal relationship of events, particularly feeding changes, illnesses, and growth faltering; (2) to control for birth weight and gestational age; and (3) to study infants who die. Longitudinal studies, following a cohort from birth or a specified age, through the period of interest, provide much better information regarding growth of that population of infants, but such studies are more expensive and often difficult to carry out in many settings in developing countries.

REVIEW OF STUDIES

Effect of Breast-feeding on Growth

Findings in low-income populations

Table V-6 summarizes studies examining feeding practices and infant growth among low-income populations. Three studies (Kanaaneh, 1972; Kanawati and McLaren, 1973; Wray and Aguirre, 1969) found breast-fed infants heavier and taller, with infants fed other foods more likely to be suffering from undernutrition. The Kanaaneh study found a dose-response relationship; as the duration and degree of breast-feeding increased, the proportion of infants in the low-weight category decreased. Other studies were inconclusive (Dugdale, 1980) or showed no difference in growth as a result of feeding method (Zeitlin et al., 1978). A study in Thailand (Viseshakul,

TABLE V-6

Studies examining the relationship between infant-feeding practices and growth:
Low-income populations

Study	Study Population	N	Conclusions
COHORT STUDY			
Venkatchalam et al., 1967	Indians	55	Mixed-fed heavier than breast-fed; no other differences in growth observed
RECONSTRUCTED COHORT STUDIES			
Kanaaneh, 1972	Arabs in Israel	610	Dose response; as duration & degree of breast-feeding rises, proportion in low-weight category falls
Dugdale, 1980	Australian aborigines	268	Inconclusive
CASE-CONTROL STUDY			
Kanawati & McLaren, 1973	Lebanese	115	Bottle-feeding in 1st 3 months associated with failure to thrive
CROSS-SECTIONAL STUDIES			
Wray & Aguirre, 1969	Colombians	213	Between ages 0–17 months, bottle-fed infants 1.5–2 times as likely to suffer from PCM[a] as breast-fed
Viseshakul, 1976	Thais	Not given	Best growth: powdered milk Good growth: tapering off at 12 months: breast milk Slower growth: sweetened condensed milk
Zeitlin et al., 1978	Filipinos	525	No differences observed

[a]Protein-calorie malnutrition

1976) found powdered milk produced the greatest growth, breast milk good growth until 12 months when growth began to taper off, and sweetened condensed milk the slowest growth. Venkatchalam et al. (1967) found mixed-fed Indian infants heavier than breast-fed infants, but observed no other growth differences. This study was the only prospective one—a controlled experiment with supplements given to one group of infants to create the mixed-feeding category.

Although much research has been devoted to studying growth of infants and children in low-income countries, few studies have compared growth in similar populations fed differently during the first year of life. Many studies are cross-sectional, and thus such important variables as birth weight and history of morbidity cannot be controlled. Few studies adequately consider morbidity effects or measure quantities of food consumed. Kanaaneh (1972) showed an association between morbidity and poor growth, but did not control for this relationship in his analysis. In supplying supplements to the infants Venkatchalam *et al.* (1967) had some measure of the quantity of food consumed in one group but no comparison measure.

Because of such methodological problems and lack of a discernible trend, the relationship between infant-feeding practices and growth is not clear. Food quantity and incidence of morbidity may be such important factors that food type alone is not a predictor of infant growth. Until a consistent relationship between food type and growth is determined, it is not possible to characterize the relationship as we did when discussing infant feeding, morbidity, and mortality. Questions of supplementation are so intimately connected to issues of quantity that they cannot be discussed separately. The questions we wish to ask are: How does mixed-feeding or supplementation affect growth? At which ages is it desirable or necessary to supplement a given feeding method? These questions can only be answered when more is known about the quantities of nutrients ingested in present infant diets and the potential variation in such quantities.

Findings in high-income populations

In high-income countries, where food supply and mother's health do not generally limit infant growth, research has focused on two issues. First, researchers have tried to evaluate the adequacy of breast milk under optimal conditions and estimate the period of time during which breast-feeding alone will promote adequate growth. Second, researchers have hypothesized that breast-feeding is adequate and less likely to lead to infantile or adolescent obesity. When less than adequate growth is found among breast-fed infants, there is a tendency to decide that the standards are inappropriate, or to interpret the findings to mean that the growth of breast-fed infants is adequate and other feeding methods lead to obesity. The two hypotheses of concern in high-income countries are (1) breast-fed infants' growth is comparable to standards used for infant growth and therefore to that of nonbreast-fed infants, and (2) nonbreast-fed infants' growth is more likely to be greater than that recommended. This amounts to the null and alternative of the one-sided hypothesis that growth of breast-fed infants will be less than or equal to that of nonbreast-fed infants.

Table V-7 summarizes studies of high-income populations. In several

TABLE V-7

Studies examining the relationship between infant-feeding practices and growth:
High-income populations

Study	Study Site & Date	N	Growth[a]	Comments
CASE SERIES STUDIES				
O'Connor, 1978	Michigan, USA	2	<	2 cases of failure to thrive on breast corrected after switching to bottle
Davies, 1979	England 1978	21	<	Examples of failure to thrive among breast-fed
Ernst et al., 1981	USA	2	<	2 cases of starvation with hypernatremic dehydration in breast-fed
Roddey et al., 1981	North Carolina, USA	4	<	4 cases of critical weight loss among breast-fed
Rowland et al., 1982	Massa-chusetts, USA	2	<	2 cases of malnutrition & hypernatremic dehydration in breast-fed
COHORT STUDIES				
Nyhan & Wessel, 1954	Connect-icut, USA	400	< at 7 days > at 6 wks	Breast-fed: wt loss greater in 1st 7 days, gain greater at 6 wks
Hodgson, 1978	England 1974−75	301	= at 6 wks, 6 mos, 1 year	No difference in wt gain at 6 wks, 6 mos, or 1 year. Earlier introduction to solids—higher mean wt at 6 mos
Dine et al., 1979	Ohio, USA	582	=	No difference in wt/ht^2, ht$\div\sqrt[3]{\text{wt}}$, wt/ht from 1 to 5 years
D'Souza & Black, 1979	England	243	>	Dose relationship with degree of supplementation: breast-fed heaviest, skinfold thickness data support wt findings
Saarinen & Siimes, 1979	Finland 1975	238	> 1st 6 mos < 6−12 mos	Breast-fed heavier 0−6 mos, lighter 6−12 mos

TABLE V-7 (continued)

Study	Study Site & Date	N	Growth[a]	Comments
COHORT STUDIES (continued)				
Ahn & MacLean, 1980	D.C.- Baltimore, Md., USA	96	= until 9 mos < after 9 mos	Growth of breast-fed similar to NCHS standards until 9 mos, when growth is less
Ferris et al., 1980	Massa- chusetts, USA	92	= until 6 mos	No difference between breast- & formula-fed during 1st 6 mos. Feeding formula plus solids before 2 months led to higher wt than feeding breast milk & food supplements
Roberts, 1980	New Zealand 1978	167	= through 5 mos	Growth similar throughout study period (5 months)
Chandra, 1982	Canada	222	= until 6 mos < after 6 mos	Growth of exclusively breast-fed similar to NCHS standards until 6 mos, when growth appears slightly lower. No statistical testing or analysis done.

[a] Growth of breast-fed infants compared to standards for infants fed other foods

studies greater growth among exclusively breast-fed infants was noted compared to standards or nonbreast-fed infants (1) at five to seven weeks (D'Souza and Black, 1979), (2) at six weeks (Nyhan and Wessel, 1954) and, (3) through six months (Saarinen and Siimes, 1979). Other studies found growth of breast-fed and nonbreast-fed or standard infants to be similar during the first five months (Chandra, 1981), to nine months (Ahn and MacLean, 1980), through the six-month study period (Ferris et al., 1980), and to the age of one year and beyond (Dine et al., 1979; S. V. Hodgson, 1978). In several cases the study period was long enough to show a change in growth of breast-fed infants relative to the standards or to the nonbreast-fed infants. Saarinen and Siimes (1979) found that although heavier during the first six months, breast-fed Finnish infants were lighter than nonbreast-fed infants during the next six months. Chandra (1981) found that after five months growth of breast-fed Canadian infants fell below the 50th percentile (NCHS, 1976) and was between the 25th and 50th percentile at six to eight months. Ahn and MacLean (1980) found growth of breast-fed U.S. infants to be comparable to NCHS standards until nine months when growth appeared to falter. Because of the short duration of exclusive breast-feeding in the U.S. and other high-income countries, sample sizes in later months become quite small. At present it appears that growth of the exclusively breast-fed infant is adequate through the first five or six months and may be so beyond that date.

If breast-fed and nonbreast-fed infants' growth is similar, higher levels of obesity in nonbreast-fed infants should not be expected. Indeed, several studies examining this issue found no association between bottle-feeding and obesity (de Swiet et al., 1977; Dubois et al., 1979; Oakley, 1977). Taitz (1971) found high levels of obesity in a group of artificially fed infants, but did not study an appropriate comparison group. These studies do not indicate that the nonbreast-fed infant is more likely to be obese than the breast-fed infant; the conclusion is that growth of the two groups is comparable.

In high-income countries both breast- and formula-feeding seem to promote growth generally considered adequate through the fifth to sixth month. After six months growth of breast-fed infants tends to be less than that of infants fed other foods. Several interpretations of these data are possible: the breast milk supply may not increase sufficiently to meet infant needs beyond a certain age; standards may not represent norms appropriate for breast-fed infants; mothers may lack the experience, awareness, and social support conducive to successful breast-feeding. The low prevalence of exclusive breast-feeding beyond age six months may preclude careful evaluation of the growth of exclusively breast-fed infants in that age group.

Several cases of severe weight loss in exclusively breast-fed upper-middle class infants appear in the literature (Davies, 1979; Ernst et al., 1981; O'Connor, 1978; Roddey et al., 1981; Rowland et al., 1982). While the numbers in each study are small (2 to 21), these studies document the possibility that failure to thrive can occur to breast-fed infants raised in conditions generally thought to be optimal. The chain of events leading to malnutrition, starvation, and the attendant clinical problems among such infants, are not understood. Because of their rarity, such cases will be difficult to study prospectively. Although it is tempting to consider such cases to result from maternal inexperience, the possibility of a physiological explanation exists and should be considered. This may indicate that breast-feeding itself is not a guarantee that the infant will receive adequate nutrition.

Effect of other foods on growth

In considering the choice of foods used to supplement or replace breast-feeding, at weaning it is important that the infant's diet approximate the ideal of a balanced diet defined by dietary recommendations. Two issues are of concern: What is the range of acceptable dietary variation within which infant growth will be adequate? What foods or combinations of foods make up diets in that acceptable range? While it is clear that a diet totally deficient in protein or particular vitamins and minerals will not be acceptable or promote adequate growth, the cutoff points between acceptable and unacceptable are not clear. Nutrient recommendations such as those of the World Health Organization (Passmore *et al.*, 1974) presently provide the main guidelines for evaluating dietary adequacy. Basic surveys are needed to catalog infant diets and describe foods used at different ages and in combination with other foods. The entire diet can then be evaluated relative to nutrient requirements. There may be a need for field studies comparing growth of infants fed these different diets, but where the diet deviates greatly from recommended intakes such studies may be unethical.

Infant diets have not yet been categorized as suggested above, and no other meaningful categorization of other foods has been developed. In the United States and England an association between early introduction of solid foods and higher weight gain and mean weight at six months has been observed (Ferris *et al.*, 1980; S. V. Hodgson, 1978). In high-income countries it is worthwhile to evaluate the calorie contribution of solid foods in infant diets. Weaning and supplemental foods are more complex issues in low-income countries because of the overall inadequacy of infant diets and the concomitant introduction of pathogens with other foods. Studies there must consider quantity and content of foods comprising the total infant diet as well as the incidence of morbidity.

CONCLUSIONS

We have evaluated some common infant foods which in early infancy may comprise the entire infant diet. In trying to evaluate adequacy of these foods, we have compared their nutritional content to dietary recommendations and the growth of breast-fed and nonbreast-fed infants to generally accepted growth standards. In each case, choice of standards is a major issue.

In evaluating effects of infant-feeding practices on growth, it seems essential to consider the amounts of foods ingested as well as their nutritional composition. At present, measuring the amounts of breast milk ingested is cumbersome; developing better low-cost measurement techniques would greatly aid research in this area. Nonetheless, we suggest that quantity of nutrients—volume of food ingested multiplied by the concentration of those nutrients in the food for each food the infant ingests during the study period—be considered when studying infant growth. All these points suggest that total infant diet be evaluated and compared with respect to infant growth and dietary recommendations. This seems the best way to evaluate the effect of infant-feeding practices on growth and to begin modifying dietary recommendations so that they more closely approach reality.

We conclude that

1. At present we do not predict infant growth differences based on differences observed in biochemical composition of infant milks. Differences may exist at the metabolic and developmental level and effects on growth will be observed later rather than in infancy. The differences may have no significant consequences or consequences cannot yet be measured. When quantity is not a major factor, as in high-income countries, growth of breast-fed and nonbreast-fed infants appears to be comparable. In low-income countries, findings are inconsistent and show no discernible trend.

2. Based on dietary recommendations, it seems that breast milk alone will promote adequate growth for two to three and possibly six months. Epidemiological evidence shows that exclusive breast-feeding in high-income settings can promote adequate growth through six months and beyond.

3. Failure to thrive or poor growth is possible on any dietary regimen if quantities fed are low. When formulas are diluted or lactation is inadequate, the infant will receive less than adequate amounts of nutrients.

6

INFANT FEEDING AND HEALTH

We discussed the effects of infant feeding on morbidity and nutritional status independently to provide a clearer understanding of each (see figure III-1). In reality, infection and nutritional status interact through various pathways to affect infant health and growth. The interaction may be synergistic. The combined presence of malnutrition and infection results in a more serious effect on the host than the sum of the effects of the two factors working independently. Alternatively, the interaction may be antagonistic; the combined effect of malnutrition and infection may be less than would be expected.

The temporal relationship between changes in nutritional status, immunocompetence, morbidity, and growth faltering are unclear. Chandra (1981) hypothesizes that inadequate nutrient intake is the first step in a chain of events leading to growth failure and impairment of immunocompetence, in turn leading to morbidity. It is equally possible that infection is the first step leading to growth faltering. How breast-feeding first affects the intervening variables nutritional status and immune status is unknown, but it is worthwhile reviewing the literature about the interaction between nutrition and infection.

EFFECTS OF NUTRITIONAL STATUS
ON RESISTANCE TO INFECTION

The synergism between nutritional deficiencies and infection operates via several pathways by which nutritional status can affect an infant's resistance to infection (see figure VI-1). The effect of nutrition on immune status has been investigated thoroughly. Deficiencies in total calories, protein, vitamins, and minerals have been shown to affect antibody production, levels of nonspecific substances such as lysozyme and interferon, and phagocytic activity, decreasing the infant's ability to resist infection and increasing

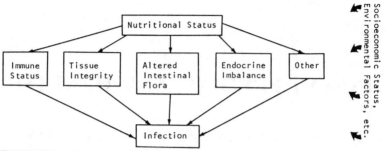

FIGURE VI-1   Effects of nutritional status on resistance to infection.

susceptibility to complications from infection (R. L. Gross and Newberne, 1980; Scrimshaw *et al.*, 1968). The exact role of these immunologic deficits in increasing susceptibility is not yet known. Rosenberg *et al.* (1976) suggest that immunologic deficits occurring in malnutrition may be irreversible among immature animals and children, thereby decreasing their ability to protect themselves from infection later in life.

Nutritional deficiencies also produce alterations in epithelial tissues which may increase susceptibility to infection, including hyperkeratosis (from vitamin A deficiency), dermatitis (riboflavin and pyridoxine deficiency), scurvy (vitamin C deficiency), and atrophy of skin or gastrointestinal mucosa (protein deficiency). It is beyond the scope of this book to discuss how specific nutrient deficiencies might increase susceptibility to infection, but it may be appropriate to give one example. Vitamin A deficiency may increase susceptibility to infection by altering immune capacity or tissue integrity (Beisel *et al.*, 1981). Scrimshaw *et al.* (1968) reviewed a number of studies in animals and humans which consistently showed strong synergism between vitamin A deficiency and infectious diseases. Unfortunately, in most studies of humans it is unclear whether the infection preceded the deficiency or vice versa, and control of other nutrients ingested is usually lacking, making a conclusion that avitaminosis A increases susceptibility to infection impossible. In animals the effect of avitaminosis A on susceptibility to infection is confirmed and evidence indicates that a deficiency of this vitamin may also alter the outcome of the infection (e.g., increase severity of the disease) (Scrimshaw *et al.*, 1968). Alterations in the gastrointestinal mucosa caused by protein-calorie or vitamin A deficiency (Scrimshaw *et al.*, 1968; Viteri and Schneider, 1974) may also alter nutrient absorption, thereby worsening nutritional status, and again increasing susceptibility to infection.

Alterations in diet may also affect quality and quantity of intestinal flora which in turn affect susceptibility to infection (Gracey *et al.*, 1974; Mata *et al.*, 1972). Malnutrition may induce flora in the gut that are normally absent, increase the number of normally nonpathogenic organisms to sufficiently high levels, induce morbidity, or displace normal flora that may be protective (Scrimshaw *et al.*, 1968). Increased levels of *lactobacillus bifidus* found in breast-fed infants may provide some protection against establishment of other harmful strains of organisms (Ross and Dawes, 1954).

Nutritional deficiencies, especially protein-calorie malnutrition, are involved in producing endocrine imbalances which make the host more susceptible to infection. A malnourished infant may produce ACTH and cortisone in abnormal amounts, which would suppress components of the immune system, making the host more susceptible (Scrimshaw *et al.*, 1968).

Antagonistic interactions between nutritional deficiencies and infection occur when a nutrient deficiency affects the infectious agent deleteriously. If certain nutrients the agent requires are deficient in the host, they may interfere with the agent's growth or multiplication; the resulting reduction in numbers of the infectious agent benefits the host.

The interaction between nutrition and infection is influenced by a variety of secondary factors (confounding variables) which may be either host or agent related, including genetic factors, sex, physiopathologic host factors, and the agent's virulence and growth requirements. None of these factors alone determines the strength and nature of the interaction; the resistance of the host, determined by genetics and environment, and the virulence of the agent act together to determine the outcome of the interaction.

Most investigations of the effect of nutritional status on infection have studied cases of severe malnutrition. Those studies do not allow determination of the effects of slight to moderate malnutrition on susceptibility to infection. Although overnutrition may also have some implications for susceptibility to infection, only the effects of undernutrition are discussed here, since in most low-income countries overnutrition is seldom a problem, and this topic is not relevant here.

EFFECTS OF INFECTION ON NUTRITIONAL STATUS

Mild and severe infections may cause nutritional deficiencies (Rosenberg *et al.*, 1976). Nutritional status may be altered via a number of pathways (see figure VI-2).

Much evidence indicates that infection is accompanied by decreased food consumption. Martorell and Yarbrough (1983) investigated food intake among 477 Guatemalan children aged one to five years. Morbidity was accompanied by an average reduction in daily intake of 175 kcal and 4.8g of protein. Several other studies had similar findings (Briscoe, 1979; Hoyle *et al.*, 1980; Mata *et al.*, 1977; Molla *et al.*, 1983; Rowland *et al.*, 1977). This decline in intake may be attributed to (1) lack of food, (2) loss of appetite, (3) physiologic inability to ingest food, (4) the mother's withdrawing solid food because of cultural beliefs and replacing it with thin gruels or liquids of poor nutritional quality, or (5) bulky diets. Withdrawal of solids is an important factor; the mother may relate a worsening diarrhea to ingestion of solid food, or believe that liquid foods may be less stressful to the infant's digestive system. The withdrawal may be based on cultural

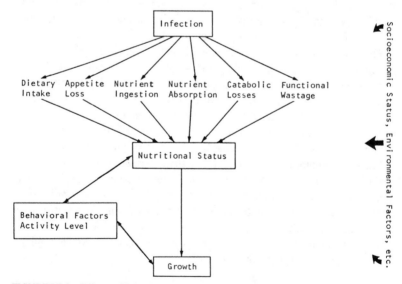

FIGURE VI-2   Effects of infection on nutritional status.

beliefs, especially in many low-income countries (Mata *et al.*, 1977; Scrimshaw *et al.*, 1968). In one study in Bangladesh, supplementary feeding decreased slightly when the child was sick with diarrhea and more pronouncedly during febrile nondiarrheal illnesses (Brown *et al.*, 1983). Hoyle *et al.* (1980) found food intake among Bangladeshi infants (16 to 22 months old) with acute diarrheal disease was significantly reduced during infection. Educational efforts to increase intake were unsuccessful. Breast-fed infants were found to be protected against reduced intake when compared to those completely weaned.

Nutrient absorption during infection may change because of clinical or subclinical infections (Briscoe, 1979; Scrimshaw *et al.*, 1968; Viteri and Schneider, 1974), further decreasing nutrients available to the body. Infestation by parasites, diarrheal disease, and use of purgatives (Scrimshaw *et al.*, 1968) are a few mechanisms that precipitate a decrease in absorption of nutrients, especially protein.

In addition to decreases in nutrient intake and nutrient absorption changes, nutritional requirements increase during infection. If these requirements are not met, and in low-income countries they usually are not, negative nutrient balance (e.g., nitrogen balance) may be expected. Nutritional costs of infection may be attributed to catabolic losses (breakdown of body tissues) or functional wastage, including loss of nutrients within the body during illness because the body is misusing them. Other costs include increased nutrient loss in body secretions, production of protective components necessary for host defense response, high nutrient costs for rebuilding damaged tissue (anabolic costs) during the recovery period, and stress.

There is considerable disagreement over the relative importance of individual pathways linking infection and nutritional status. The major issue appears to be the relative importance of the metabolic and behavioral effects of infection. Little information is available on each pathway and no study has examined them all. Moreover, since behavioral pathways are culturally specific, the relative importance of behavioral and biological pathways varies greatly across cultures. Only Briscoe (1979) has tried to review the quantitative importance of all these pathways which may link infection and nutritional status. He suggests:

1. Nitrogen loss may be overestimated because possible decrease in activity during infection is not considered in calculations of requirements during infection, or the amount of muscle protein going to gluconeogenesis (production of energy from noncarbohydrate sources) may be overestimated.

2. Malabsorption of nutrients may be incorrectly estimated, with no severe alterations expected during infection.

3. Catabolic losses are quantitatively dependent on severity and duration of fever during illness.

Data from Briscoe's cohort study in Bangladesh among children from birth to age five, used to estimate components of food lost because of subclinical infection, indicated that anorexia and food withdrawal were the main factors contributing to possible deterioration in nutritional status.

Deterioration in nutritional status during periods of normally rapid growth is expected to result in weight loss and decreased growth in height (Scrimshaw *et al.*, 1968). Poor nutritional status may be expressed by poor growth, apathy, and lowered activity levels. Behavioral interchange between mother and infant may be affected. A thin, slight child who is inactive may not stimulate a mother to feed, hold, or interact with it in other ways. The child will probably be less demanding and consequently be fed less often than a more demanding and active child. The nutritional status and growth of this less active child may then deteriorate further (Cravioto, 1972; Cravioto and Delicardi, 1976).

CONCLUSIONS

The various factors affecting infant health are clearly closely intertwined, reacting with each other in a cyclical manner. Nutritional status and infection interact to affect health more or less severely depending on the individual's resistance and the virulence of the infectious agent. For an infant with poor nutritional status, the outcome of an infection may be severe and accompanied by complications. During the recovery period, nutritional anabolic requirements are extremely high. An infant lacking adequate nutrient intake during recovery from infection will be extremely susceptible to reinfection; thus begins the cyclical pattern of infection and deteriorating nutritional status.

It is difficult to study the temporality of events in the nutritional status-infection relationship. Available data do not indicate whether infection or poor nutritional state initiates the cycle which ultimately affects infant health. According to Waterlow (1981, p. 95), "there is evidence from several countries that the peak prevalence of diarrhoeal disease occurs after growth has begun to fall off." Further research is needed, particularly longitudinal studies of the onset and history of infection and nutritional status. To delineate the behavioral effects of infection on nutritional status, investigations of family food consumption patterns and beliefs are needed. The relative quantitative importance of the pathways in figures VI-1 and VI-2 requires further investigation.

Finally, it is important to reiterate that discussing intervening variables independent of each other is artificial since in reality there is a great deal of interaction. As a matter of convenience in testing specific hypotheses, we discuss these factors separately as they affect infant health and growth.

7

INFANT FEEDING
AND MATERNAL NUTRITION

While infant feeding has its most obvious impact on the infant's health, it also affects the mother. In chapters 7 and 8 we discuss two significant impacts of infant feeding on the mother: effects on her nutritional status and her fecundity and fertility.

NUTRITIONAL STATUS

Theoretical Pathways

Maternal nutritional status results from a complex interplay of factors which can be influenced by choice of infant-feeding method (figure VII-1). Three primary factors—dietary intake, its absorption and use, and maternal nutrient stores—determine the availability of nutrients to the mother. Other factors—basal metabolic rate, level of breast milk production, physical activity, and physiologic losses—determine her metabolic needs. Ultimately, if the woman is to survive, a balance must be achieved between metabolic needs and availability of nutrients. How that balance is achieved may affect her nutritional status.

If food supplies are inadequate to meet maternal metabolic needs—a situation common in developing countries—compensatory social and biological responses may be initiated which increase availability of nutrients or decrease needs. A mother may decrease her nutrient needs by decreasing her physical activity, which may affect her ability to earn an income. Alternatively, the volume of breast milk a mother with inadequate intakes produces may be low enough to endanger her infant's nutritional health. These potential adaptive responses may maintain maternal levels of common indicators of nutritional status such as weight and hemoglobin. However,

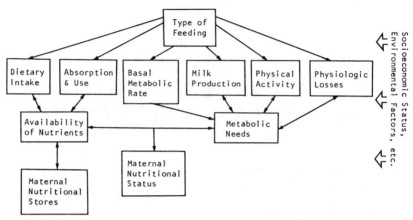

FIGURE VII-1   Effects of infant feeding on maternal nutritional status.

using a broad definition of nutritional status, the mother's inability to fulfill her expected social and biological functions adequately as an income generator or provider of breast milk indicates that her nutritional status is suboptimal.

Other adaptive mechanisms may directly affect maternal nutritional status indicators. If exogenous nutrient supplies are inadequate, maternal stores may be called on to fill the gap. Whether this use of stored nutrients impairs nutritional status depends on the level of maternal stores and the severity and duration of the deficit. Most healthy individuals, such as well-nourished lactating women, have a reservoir of nutrients, especially calories, which can be used temporarily without harm to their nutritional health. However, if initial stores are low or nonexistent, as in the chronically undernourished mother, or the deficit is great or of long duration, the continued use of stores will lead to impaired nutritional status, manifested by clinically defined deficiency syndromes.

The potential effects of breast-feeding on maternal nutritional status are obvious. Lactation may prompt a mother voluntarily to increase her food intake. Hytten and Leitch (1971) offer some evidence that physiological changes brought about by lactation may improve a woman's absorption and use of ingested nutrients. A lactating woman's metabolic needs are primarily affected by the nutrient cost of producing breast milk. Some compensation may be achieved by a lower basal metabolic rate and a reduction in normal nutrient losses such as reduced iron losses because of delay in return of menstruation, and by an enhanced efficiency in energy production (Whitehead, 1983). A more significant compensation may be achieved by reduced physical activity.

The potential effects on maternal nutritional status of feeding infants foods other than breast milk are not as obvious, but can theoretically be significant, especially in developing countries. The cost of providing breast milk substitutes may mean that less money is available for food for the mother, resulting in a decrease in the quantity and quality of food she consumes.

Feeding the infant other foods will of course not produce maternal physiological changes in absorption and use of nutrients, basal metabolic rate, or physiologic losses. Physical activity may be affected if the cost of providing other foods forces a mother to spend more time in market labor, thus changing her activity patterns.

Cultural practices may have an impact on factors affecting the nutritional status of lactating or postpartum women. There are many culturally determined avoidances of certain foods by pregnant or lactating women (Katona-Apte, 1977; Sundararaj and Pereira, 1975; Wellin, 1955). Sundararaj and Pereira (1975) found dietary intakes at 4 weeks of lactation in India considerably worse than at 16 weeks, presumably because of the influence of food taboos during the early weeks. McGuire (1979) described a sequence of restrictions in physical activity imposed on postpartum women in rural Guatemala which could affect their energy needs. In a review of anthropological studies on postpartum cultural practices in 195 preindustrial societies, Jimenez and Newton (1979) found in nearly half the societies, postpartum women customarily returned to their usual duties within two weeks of delivery. On the other hand, in 12 percent of the cultures, postpartum women were normally allowed over two months of rest after childbirth before resuming their usual activities.

Methodological Issues

Outcome variable—Indicators of nutritional status

The usual indicators of nutritional status are dietary intake data, anthropometric and biochemical measurements, clinical signs and symptoms. A complete assessment of nutritional status should consider all these indicators but time and money usually restrict a study to fewer measures. More complete discussions of the advantages and disadvantages of various assessment techniques are available (Austin, 1978; Christakis, 1973; Hamilton *et al.*, 1984).

Dietary intake is one of the more common indicators used for assessing nutritional status, despite problems with the accuracy of current data collection techniques (Acheson *et al.*, 1980; Christakis, 1977; Pekkerinen, 1970; Young *et al.*, 1952). Dietary intake, however, is one determinant of nutritional status, not a direct measure of it. Dietary adequacy depends on several other factors—use of ingested nutrients, current maternal stores, overall nutritional needs—all highly individual and interrelated. Most nutritional assessments relate dietary intakes to some officially recommended intake level. The method most commonly used to characterize a population's intake is to determine mean intakes relative to recommended levels. Because of the way recommended intakes are derived (NRC, 1980), means are not useful in evaluating the degree to which a group suffers from inadequate intakes. Actual mean nutrient intakes below the recommended levels do not necessarily indicate an inadequate diet, nor do such figures provide information on the percentage of the population who may be at risk. A low mean intake suggests dietary insufficiency, but is by no means conclusive.

Table VII-1 gives current recommendations on adequate dietary intakes for lactating women, as determined by the World Health Organization. Difficulties of arriving at recommendations for one specific population group are great. Deriving recommendations for widely diverse cultural groups is even more difficult. Current recommendations reflect the current body of knowledge, which is far from complete and surrounded by considerable controversy, primarily because of assumptions made concerning underlying determinants of nutritional needs, which may not be true for lactating women in developing countries (Beaton, 1979; Jelliffe and Jelliffe, 1978b; U.N. University, 1979; Whitehead, 1979). Whitehead (1983) discusses thoroughly the current state of knowledge about nutrient requirements of lactating women in developing countries.

Some of the assumptions made in formulating these recommendations may result in underestimating the dietary needs of lactating women in developing countries. The recommendations are based on data from healthy, well-nourished Caucasian women engaged in light to moderate activity. The typical Third World woman may be in ill health, chronically malnourished, and engaged in strenuous physical activity. The recommendations are based on a mixed diet rich in animal foods whereas Third World women generally consume little food of animal origin (Hamilton *et al.*, 1984). They assume an adequate weight gain during pregnancy, with deposition of about 4 kg of fat, equivalent to approximately 36,000 kcal. Women

TABLE VII-1

Recommended daily nutrient intakes for women—World Health Organization, 1974

	Adult (moderately active)	Pregnant (later half)	Lactating (1st 6 mos)
Energy (kcal)	2200.0	+350.0	+550.0
Protein (g)[a]	29.0	38.0	46.0
Vitamin A (μg)	750.0	750.0	1200.0
Vitamin D (μg)	2.5	10.0	10.0
Thiamin (mg)	0.9	+0.1	+0.2
Riboflavin (mg)	1.3	+0.2	+0.4
Niacin (mg)	14.5	+2.3	+3.7
Folic Acid (μg)	200.0	400.0	300.0
Vitamin B_{12} (μg)	2.0	3.0	2.5
Vitamin C (mg)	30.0	50.0	50.0
Calcium (g)	0.4−0.5	1.0−1.2	1.0−1.2
Iron (mg)	14−28.0	14−28.0[b]	14−28.0[a]

Source: Passmore et al., 1974

[a]As egg or milk protein

[b]For women with inadequate iron status at beginning of pregnancy, requirement is increased.

in developing countries generally experience low weight gains during pregnancy (Hytten, 1964; Rajalakshmi, 1971; Schutz et al., 1980). Hytten (1964) calculated that at weight gains of 6.5 kg and a birth weight of 2.9 kg, only 1 kg of fat is stored during pregnancy. He postulated that storage may take place during early pregnancy and the stored fat would probably be used to meet increased energy needs during the latter half of pregnancy rather than being available during lactation. Current recommendations note that lactating women who have experienced low weight gains during pregnancy should consume more calories.

Other assumptions may result in an overestimate of the needs of lactating women in developing countries. Current recommendations assume that breast milk is produced at an efficiency level of 80 percent, that is, it takes 100 kcal of additional food for the mother to produce 80 kcal of breast milk. Thomson et al. (1970) indicates that the efficiency may be as high as 90 percent. The recommendations are based on an average production of 850 ml of milk per day, which Jelliffe and Jelliffe (1978b) claim is an arbitrary figure, based on 1950 assumptions by the U.N. Committee on Calorie Requirements. Using multiple regression analysis, Whitehead and Paul (1981) predicted breast milk requirements of healthy, fully breast-fed

British infants growing along the 50th percentile of the NCHS standards and found that the required energy intake was 15 to 20 percent below the WHO recommendations. The recommended figure is certainly higher than actual average production by women studied in developing countries (Jelliffe and Jelliffe, 1978b; Whitehead, 1979). Whether the low breast milk output of many Third World women is physiologically normal and adequate for infant growth and development or is an adaptation to inadequate dietary intakes is not known. Finally, there is growing evidence that lactating women in developing countries may absorb and use nutrients more efficiently than do women in developed countries (Coward *et al.*, 1984; Prentice *et al.*, 1981; Whitehead, 1983).

Anthropometric measurements most appropriate to the assessment of the effect of infant feeding on maternal nutritional status are changes in weight (controlled for height) and in body composition, including skinfold thicknesses and arm muscle circumference. Because of possible accumulation of fat stores during pregnancy, some reduction in weight and skinfold thicknesses would be expected to occur in mothers after childbirth. Taggert *et al.* (1967) have shown among a group of well-nourished women in Scotland that skinfold thicknesses increased during pregnancy primarily in the abdomen, back, and upper thighs. Similar studies have not been conducted on poorly nourished Third World women. If all fat stored during pregnancy is lost during subsequent lactation, no significant change would be expected in other measures of skinfold thickness, such as triceps. If changes do occur in triceps skinfold thickness, stores laid down during pregnancy may be depleted and other maternal stores are being used, at possible risk to the mother.

Biochemical measures of nutritional status include hemoglobin, hematocrit, and other measures of iron status, plasma and tissue levels of nutrients, and tests of functional capacity of the body's stores of nutrients, for example, level of activity of enzyme systems which require certain vitamins in order to function. A full assessment of the effect of infant feeding on these biochemical indicators should include comparison of actual values to standards and changes in values over time.

While clinical indicators of nutritional status may be useful in identifying and treating individual cases of malnutrition, their value in field surveys and epidemiologic studies is limited. Many clinical symptoms are not specific to nutritional deficiencies nor are they sensitive to marginal changes in nutritional status. In addition, recognition of symptoms is somewhat subjective, leading to a lack of agreement among different observers. Clinical symptoms may be used as clues to possible nutrient deficiencies, but should always be accompanied by more definitive assessment techniques (Christakis, 1973).

To determine the effect of infant feeding on maternal nutritional status, these indicators should be measured over time. If indicators are measured only at one point, results could be misleading. For instance, lactating women may, at a given time, weigh less than nonlactating, postpartum women. Because of weight gains during pregnancy, it is not clear that lower weights of lactating women are detrimental unless it can be shown that they have lost more weight than could be accounted for by fat stores laid down during pregnancy.

Exposure variable – Infant feeding

Specification of the independent variable, method of feeding, should be in terms of some measure of the quantity of food supplied by breast-feeding or other foods. For a lactating woman, the actual quantity of nutrients lost in the process of producing breast milk may most dramatically affect her nutritional status. Since the caloric and possibly protein density of breast milk appear to be fairly stable (see chapter 5) and the energy cost of producing breast milk is related to the volume produced, quantity of calories and protein the mother loses can be calculated from measures or estimates of the volume of milk produced. The density of other nutrients may vary more, and an accurate measure of the cost to the mother requires a knowledge not only of the quantity of milk an individual woman produces, but of its specific nutrient density as well.

Since the effect on a mother's nutritional status of feeding infants other foods is likely to be experienced through a reduction in the availability of food because of the cost of breast milk substitutes, the actual cost of feeding other foods may be a more appropriate measure than the volume of substitutes fed. Similar volumes of other foods can have dramatically different costs depending on form of the substitute, where it was purchased, and quantities purchased.

Confounding variables

A host of variables may independently affect choice of feeding method and determinants of maternal nutritional status and must be controlled for in any study. For a detailed discussion, see Hamilton et al. (1984). Socio-economic status is perhaps the most obvious and strongest. The mother's work status can affect her choice of feeding method and level of physical activity, and thus her nutritional needs. Similarly, mother's health status can affect choice of feeding method and nutritional needs. Since type of feeding method may affect fertility, pregnancy status—affecting nutritional needs—may differ in lactating versus nonlactating women (at the same time postpartum, a nonlactating woman may be more likely to be pregnant than a nursing mother). It is important, therefore, to control for pregnancy in any analysis.

REVIEW OF STUDIES

Tables VII-2 through VII-5 summarize a number of studies conducted on nutritional status of lactating women in developing countries. Most of this research focused on indicators of nutritional status of lactating women, not on evaluating the effects of lactation on these indicators or on other components of a broader definition of nutritional health, such as physical activity. No studies have evaluated the effects of other feeding methods on maternal health. Several studies provide nutritional status indicators for lactating women without a comparison group. With such limited information, findings of poor nutritional status cannot be attributed to lactation since all women in a country, regardless of lactational status, may be poorly nourished. Other studies have compared values for lactating women with those for nonpregnant, nonlactating women. Unless the latter group is composed of women at a similar stage postpartum to the lactating women, differences could be because of biological and social factors affecting the nutritional status of all postpartum women, regardless of whether they are lactating. A similar problem arises in comparing values of lactating women with their own prepregnant values. Changes found may be because of their postpartum state, rather than lactation.

Other methodological problems limit the validity of conclusions drawn from these studies. Samples in most studies are relatively small and nonrepresentative. Of studies using various types of nutritional status indicators, few have applied more than one indicator to a population, making it difficult to attribute results to dietary deficiencies alone. When comparisons are made, statistical analyses are rarely performed which would evaluate the significance of differences found. Finally, confounding variables, such as socioeconomic status, are not usually adequately controlled for.

TABLE VII-2

Caloric and protein intake of lactating women vs. pregnant and nonpregnant, nonlactating women, and dietary recommendations

Study	Sample/Study Characteristics	Daily Caloric Intake				Daily Protein Intake (g)			
		Mean	LW/PW[1] × 100	LW/NPNL[2] × 100	LW/DR[3] × 100	Mean	LW/PW[1] × 100	LW/NPNL[2] × 100	LW/DR[3] × 100
AFRICA									
Paul et al.[9,a] 1979b, Gambia	LW (0–7 mos): 33[4]								
	Mar.–Jun.	1740	107.4		63.3				
	Jul.–Oct.	1370	103.1		49.8				
	Nov.–Dec.	1890	133.1		68.7				
	PW (same women): 33[5]								
	Mar.–Jun.	1620							
	Jul.–Oct.	1340							
	Nov.–Dec.	1420							
Paul & Müller[4,a,b] 1980, Gambia	LW: 31 Aug.					35	83.3		76.0
	PW: 31 (same) Nov.					68	125.9		147.8
ASIA									
Pasricha[10,b,c] 1958, India	LW: 70[6] PW: 100 NPNL: same subjects	1858	102.4	86.3	67.6	42.7	97.0	85.7	92.8
Karmarkar et al.[10,a] 1959, India	LW: very poor (N = 54)[6] prepregnant	1439			52.3	39.6			86.1
	poor (N = 50)	1872			68.1	46.1			100.2
	middle (N = 57)	1906			69.3	47.2			119.6
	upper middle (N = 49)	2279			82.9	55.0			119.6

TABLE VII-2 (continued)

Study	Sample/Study Characteristics	Daily Caloric Intake				Daily Protein Intake (g)			
		Mean	LW/PW[1] × 100	LW/NPNL[2] × 100	LW/DR[3] × 100	Mean	LW/PW[1] × 100	LW/NPNL[2] × 100	LW/DR[3] × 100
Devadas & Mangalam[10,a] 1970, India	LW: 24 Low SES[4]	1524			58.6	39.0			60.0
Devadas et al.[b] 1971, India	LW: supplemented: N = 12[4]	1515			52.2	54.0			83.1
	controls: N = 12	1399			50.9	39.0			60.0
Sundararaj & Pereira[b] 1975, India	LW: 39 4 wks[6]	1702			83.8	35.0			63.6
	16 wks	2090			102.9	42.6			77.4
	52 wks	1711			84.2	35.6			64.7
Villa-Real[b] 1975, Philippines	LW: 21[7]	2175			75.0	66.0			88.0
Nutrition Foundation of the Philippines[b] 1977, Philippines	LW: 74[8] PW: 39	1599 1591	100.5		65.6	49.0 54.0	90.7		63.0
Devadas et al.[b] 1978, India	LW: 20[4]	2961			102.1	65.0			100.0
Durnin[11,12,b] 1980, New Guinea	Coastal: LW < 1 yr: 13[4]	1412	99.8	100.7	51.3	24.1	94.9	104.3	52.4
	LW > 1 yr: 19	1491				27.7			
	PW: 9	1414				25.4			
	NPNL: 14	1402				23.1			
	Highland: LW < 1 yr: 14	2133	106.6	101.3	77.6	43.0	93.7	98.6	93.5
	LW > 1 yr: 6	2247				39.6			
	PW: 7	2001				45.9			
	NPNL: 14	2105				43.6			

TABLE VII-2 (continued)

Study	Sample/Study Characteristics	Daily Caloric Intake				Daily Protein Intake (g)			
		Mean	LW/PW[1] × 100	LW/NPNL[2] × 100	LW/DR[3] × 100	Mean	LW/PW[1] × 100	LW/NPNL[2] × 100	LW/DR[3] × 100
Rajalakshmi[4,5,g] 1980, India	LW (low income): 50	1620			80.1–90.0	58.0			126.0
	LW (upper income): 18	2020			96.0–110.0	54.0			
LATIN AMERICA Arroyave[b] 1976, Guatemala	LW: 36[8]	1599	87.9	112.8	67.0	58.0	107.4	148.7	126.0
	PW 3rd trimester: 57	1819				54.0			
Chávez & Martínez,[7,b,h]	NPNL (PW, 1st trimester): 20	1418				39.0			
1980, Mexico	LW (6th month): 17	2040	104.6		74.2	53.3	106.4		115.9
Schutz et al.[c]	PW (same, 4th month): 17	1950				50.1			
1980, Guatemala	LW: 18[8]	1929		102.8	70.1	47.6		118.4	103.5
Delgado et al.[3,11,b,d]	NPNL: 6	1876							
1981, Guatemala	Both groups supplemented								
	LW: N (unknown)[8]								
	Supplemented 3 mos	1766			68.9	55.5			90.6
	6 mos	1764			69.8	55.2			91.3
	9 mos	1795			72.1	54.5			91.3
	12 mos	1708			69.4	54.0			91.3
Valverde et al.[4,11]	N = 107–333[7]								
1981, Guatemala	LW: 3–9 mos	2320–	113.2–		84.4–				
		2400			87.3				
	12–15 mos	2200–	117.1						
	PW: 1st half	2275							
	2nd half	2150							
		2050							
MIDDLE EAST Geissler et al.[8,10,f]	LW (3 months)								
1978, Iran	Low SES: 21	1840			70	61			90
	Middle SES: 36	2270			80	82			120

Notes: *Ratio of mean intakes of lactating women &* (1) pregnant women; (2) nonpregnant, nonlactating women; (3) recommended intake

Measurement technique: (4) weighed food records; (5) lab analysis of cooked food sample; (6) questionnaire; (7) unknown; (8) 24-hr recalls

Controlled variables: (9) season; (10) socioeconomic status; (11) lactation duration; (12) residence; (13) wt; (14) baby's sex; (15) income

Comments: (a) Difference LW–PW in Nov.–Dec. statistically significant at p<0.01; LW in July–Oct. vs Nov.–Dec. significant at p<0.001; (b) no statistical tests; (c) data on NPNL collected retrospectively; (d) not representative of unsupplemented intake; (e) no significant difference in calorie, protein, supplement intake between LW and NPNL; (f) significant difference between socioeconomic groups; (g) author's calculations of requirements used; (h) mildly malnourished.

TABLE VII-3

Vitamin and mineral intakes of lactating women in low-income countries

Study	Vitamins A	C	Riboflavin	Thiamin	Niacin	Iron	Calcium
AFRICA: Gambia							
Paul & Müller, 1980			D	A	A		
Whitehead et al., 1981	D		D				D
Bates et al., 1981			D				
Bates et al., 1982	A (May–June) D (July–April)						
ASIA: India							
Pasricha, 1958						A	D
Karmarkar et al., 1959						A	D
Devadas & Mangalam, 1970	D	D	D	D		D	D
Devadas et al., 1971	D	D		D		A	D
Sundararaj & Pereira, 1975	D	D	D	A	D	A	D
Devadas et al., 1978	D	D	D	A		D	D
ASIA: Philippines							
Villa-Real, 1975	D	D	D	D	A	D	D
Nutrition Foundation of the Philippines, 1977	D	D	D	D	D	D	D
LATIN AMERICA: Guatemala							
Arroyave, 1976	D	D	D	A		A	D
MIDDLE EAST: Iran							
Geissler et al., 1978	A[a]	A	D	A		D	D
	D[b]	A	D	A		D	D

Notes: A = adequate intake; mean intake above WHO recommended level
D = deficient intake; mean intake below WHO recommended level
[a]middle socioeconomic status; [b]low socioeconomic status

TABLE VII-4

Biochemical indicators of nutritional status of lactating women (LW) in developing countries

Study	Sample	Vitamin A (serum retinol)	Riboflavin (enzyme activity)	Iron	Calcium (serum levels)	Comments
AFRICA Fenuku & Earl-Quarcoo, 1978 Ghana	Low SES: LW (7 wks– 6 mos): 36 NPNL: 28				Significantly lower in LW vs NPNL but within normal limits	No intake data
Thein, 1979 Ethiopia		40% LW deficient serum retinol (< 10 µg/100 ml)				Author claims generally adequate intakes among Ethiopians but gives no data
Bates et al., 1981 Gambia	LW		$\overline{X}$ EGRAC = 1.82 (at risk)			Low intakes; EGRAC significantly higher than in healthy British LW
ASIA: India Devadas & Mangalam, 1970	LW in village with nutrition program: 24			79% anemic		"Reasonably adequate intake"

TABLE VII-4 (continued)

Study	Sample	Vitamin A (serum retinol)	Riboflavin (enzyme activity)	Iron	Calcium (serum levels)	Comments
ASIA: India (continued)						
Devadas et al., 1971	LW; supplemented: 12			$\overline{X}$ initial Hgb = 10.7 (at risk) final = 11.91		$\overline{X}$ intake-supplemented: 34 mg controls: 37mg both adequate
	Controls: 12			$\overline{X}$ initial Hgb = 10.87 (at risk) final = 11.11		
Rajalakshmi, 1971	Unknown	No change from parturition to 6 mos lactation		Hgb: no change from parturition to 6 mos lactation	No change from parturition to 6 mos lactation	Gives no data; initial values low; intakes adequate
Devadas et al., 1978	LW: 20	Serum retinol		Hgb: 74% < 12 g/100 ml (at risk)		Intake inadequate
	LW: 10 mg	$\overline{X}$ = 49 µg/100 ml (adequate)				$\overline{X}$ intake = 28

TABLE VII-4 (continued)

Study	Sample	Vitamin A (serum retinol)	Riboflavin (enzyme activity)	Iron	Calcium (serum levels)	Comments
ASIA: India (continued)						
Prema et al., 1981	Low SES, CP:			Hgb: $\overline{X}$		
	NPNL: 1025					
	LW < 6 mos: 784			11.7		
	LW 7–12 mos: 560			12.2		
	LW > 12 mos: 652			11.9		
				11.6		
	Low SES, FPP:					
	NPNL: 642					
	LW < 6 mos: 422			12.6		
	LW 7–12 mos: 486			12.8		
	LW > 12 mos: 429			12.7		
				12.5		
LATIN AMERICA: Guatemala						
Schutz et al., 1980	LW avg 10 mos postpartum: 18			Hgb: $\overline{X}$=13.3 Hct: $\overline{X}$=39		No information on dietary intake
	NPNL: 6			Hgb: $\overline{X}$=13.6 Hct: $\overline{X}$=39		
MIDDLE EAST: Iran						
Geissler et al., 1978	LW, middle SES			Hgb: $\overline{X}$=13.3 Hct: $\overline{X}$=40		
	LW, low SES			Hgb: $\overline{X}$=10.8 Hct: $\overline{X}$=38		

Notes: CP = clinic patients; FPP = family planning patients; NPNL = nonpregnant, nonlactating; SES = socioeconomic status.
Information on vitamin C (serum levels) available only in Bates *et al.*, 1982; LW had lower levels than PW or NPNL: 1.2 mg/dl in May–June, 0.2 ml/dl in Sept.–Oct.

TABLE VII-5

Anthropometric indicators of nutritional status of lactating women (LW)
in developing countries

Study	Sample	Weight (wt)	Skinfold Thickness	Comments
AFRICA: Gambia				
Thomson et al., 1966	LW 4–36 wks: 62 longitudinal NPNL: 14	Rainy season: wt loss in both LW & NPNL; other seasons: LW maintained or gained wt		Indicates competition between replenishing maternal stores & milk production
Paul et al., 1979b	LW thru 3 mos: 29	Rainy season: wt loss; other seasons: gained, even at low intakes	Rainy season: reduced triceps & subscapular; otherwise, increase	
ASIA				
Devadas et al., 1971 India	LW supplement: 12 controls: 12	$\overline{X}$ wt loss = 1.79 kg $\overline{X}$ wt loss = 2.91 kg		No comparison with prepregnant wts
Devadas et al., 1978 India	LW: 40 longitudinal over 6 mos lactation	Teenage: LW lost 1.4 kg Adult: LW lost 0.3 kg		No comparison with prepregnant wts
Harrison et al., 1975 New Guinea	LW: 153	Wt & ponderal index (ht $\div$ $\sqrt[3]{wt}$) significant & negatively associated with lactation duration	Not significantly related to lactation duration	No comparison with prepregnant values
Kusin et al., 1979 East Java	LW: 1369	23% wt/ht < 90%ile 35% wt/ht < 90%ile		Unclear if lactation leads to better nutrition or if better nourished mothers more likely to lactate

TABLE VII-5 (continued)

Study	Sample	Weight (wt)	Skinfold Thickness	Comments
LATIN AMERICA: Guatemala				
Delgado et al., 1981	LW: 480–552 supplemented	Vs 1st-trimester women, LW at 12 mos lost 0.90 kg (−7.14 kg during lactation)		Unclear if study cross-sectional or longitudinal; no data on unsupplemented LW
Schutz et al., 1980	LW: 18 (avg 10 mos PP) NPNL: 6(avg 26 mos PP)	Losing avg 369 g/mo Losing 35 g/mo no significant difference in LW & NPNL wts		No comparison with prepregnant wts; wt loss rate differences may be due to different times pp
Valverde et al., 1981	LW: 251–272	Wt loss in 1st 12 mos lactation but not below wt in 1st half of pregnancy		No data on prepregnant wts

Notes: NPNL = nonpregnant nonlactating; PP = postpartum

Dietary Intake

Table VII-2 summarizes results of studies of calorie and protein intake of lactating women in low-income countries. Most studies have found inadequate dietary intakes when compared with recommendations, with deficiencies in calories generally more prevalent and more severe than protein deficiencies. Calorie recommendations for lactation were met in only two cases, in India (Devadas *et al.*, 1978; Sundararaj and Pereira, 1975). In several studies, lactating women were consuming approximately half the recommended level of calories; deficiencies were often in the range of 1,000 kcal. Lactating women generally increased their caloric intakes only slightly over those of their nonpregnant, nonlactating counterparts, whose diets were already deficient in calories. These low intake figures may be the result of systematic biases in the measurement techniques. That similar results were found using a variety of techniques for measuring dietary intakes suggests, however, that measurement bias has not had a major impact on the findings.

A series of detailed studies has been conducted on lactating women in the Gambia to determine the consequences of a diet seemingly highly deficient in energy. During the dry season, a time of relative abundance, energy intakes of lactating women in the first three months postpartum averaged 1,773 kcal/day, nearly 300 kcal/day more than during pregnancy (Prentice, 1980; Prentice *et al.*, 1981). However, during the rainy season, a time of depleted food stores and heavy agricultural labor prior to the harvest, energy intakes of lactating women reached a minimum mean level of 1,203 kcal/a day, significantly lower than the intake of pregnant women during the same season. Although the dry season intake was approximately a thousand calories below WHO recommendations, these lactating women produced enough breast milk for adequate infant growth for the first three months, did not appear to lower their physical activity, and even managed to gain an average of 0.59 kg/month. However, during the severe food restrictions of the wet season, the lactating women lost weight (an average of −0.74 kg/month), produced less breast milk, and their infants had a more difficult time maintaining adequate growth (Prentice *et al.*, 1981).

Combining information on energy intake, weight changes, and breast milk output (assuming an 80 percent conversion efficiency), Prentice *et al.* (1981) calculated the residual energy of lactating women, defined as the amount of energy available for basal metabolic rate (BMR) and activity, and found it remarkably similar in both seasons (1,033 kcal/day during the dry season and 1,070 kcal/day during the wet season), but well below most calculations of BMR alone. (The authors mention a range in BMR calculations from 1,155 kcal/day to 1,339 kcal/day). Prentice and colleagues conclude that an energy intake of 1,770 kcal/day may be adequate, at least for the first three months of lactation, to maintain infant and maternal health in the Gambia; the discrepancy between this figure and WHO recommendations may be because of a higher level of metabolic efficiency among Gambian women.

Subsequent supplementation studies on the same women revealed that increasing their average energy intake to 2,291 kcal/day and eliminating the sharp decrease in energy intake during the rainy season did not have dramatic effects on infant or maternal health. Supplemented women were one to two kg heavier than unsupplemented controls, but still lost weight during the rainy season despite an average increase in energy intake of 1,100 kcal/day. There was no significant change in breast milk output. Anecdotal information indicates that supplemented women worked harder, but no data on energy expenditure during physical activity were presented. The percentage of women reporting being "totally well" increased from 40 percent to 62 percent after the supplement (Coward et al., 1984). The authors suggest that the energy supplement brought about a decrease in the efficiency of energy conversion, but such conclusions cannot be substantiated without data on the effect of supplementation on physical activity. If supplementation did bring about an increase in physical activity, it would suggest that while a presupplementation intake of 1,770 kcal may be adequate for maternal and infant health, it is not necessarily optimal.

Rajalakshmi (1980) calculated energy requirements of low-income and upper income lactating Indian women and found them to be substantially lower than WHO recommendations. Despite the low intake, there was no significant maternal weight loss after six months of breast-feeding.

Protein intakes more often met the requirements, although it must be kept in mind that when caloric intakes are inadequate, protein is likely to be used for energy. Also, the quality of protein of typical Third World diets is generally lower than the high-quality egg and milk protein on which recommendations are based (Hamilton et al., 1984). Geissler et al. (1978) compared protein intakes of middle and low-income lactating women in Iran to a theoretical requirement of 65 g (corrected for the low protein quality of a diet of mixed animal and vegetable protein) and found both groups were consuming adequate amounts. Only in coastal New Guinea were intakes as low as half the requirement. Protein intakes of lactating New Guinea women were generally slightly lower than those of pregnant women, whereas caloric intakes were slightly higher, indicating a possible shift in the pattern of food consumption toward more starchy, lower protein items. In studies comparing protein intake of lactating women to that of nonpregnant, nonlactating women, lactating women generally consumed the same amount or slightly more protein (Arroyave, 1976; Durnin, 1980; NFP, 1977; Pasricha, 1958; Schutz et al., 1980).

Table VII-3 summarizes studies on the adequacy of vitamin and mineral intakes by lactating women (as compared with current WHO recommendations). For simplicity's sake, mean intakes were considered deficient if they fell below the current recommended level and adequate if above. In all the studies surveyed, the diets of lactating women were deficient in vitamins A and C, riboflavin, and calcium, and in most studies the deficiencies were large. Thiamine intakes were deficient in half the studies and niacin was deficient in two-thirds. Iron intake was adequate in half the studies and inadequate (although only marginally so) in the remaining half.

Biochemical Indices

In table VII-4 we summarize the findings of studies on biochemical indices of nutritional status of lactating women. Since results for any one nutrient are inconsistent, no overall generalizations are possible. The iron status of lactating women has been most frequently assessed using hemoglobin and hematocrit levels. In India, Devadas and colleagues (Devadas and Mangalam, 1970; Devadas et al., 1971, 1978) found a high proportion of women with anemia based on hemoglobin measurements, although mean intakes of iron appeared adequate. On the other hand, Schutz et al. (1980) found adequate mean hemoglobin and hematocrit levels among lactating women in Guatemala with no differences compared to nonpregnant, nonlactating controls.

Among low-income women in India, Prema et al. (1981) found a rise in hemoglobin during the first six months of lactation as compared with nonpregnant nonlactating women, with a decline thereafter. Hemoglobin values for women who had been breast-feeding more than 12 months were not significantly different than those for nonpregnant, nonlactating women. Prema and colleagues speculated that the rise in hemoglobin during the early stages of lactation is a physiologically normal consequence of changes in the hemopoietic system during pregnancy and would therefore be expected to occur in both lactating and nonlactating, postpartum women. Further studies comparing lactating women with nonlactating, postpartum women are necessary to clarify this issue.

Despite the prevalence of inadequate dietary calcium intakes among lactating women in developing countries, there is no biochemical evidence that lactation itself adversely affects indicators of calcium status. Widdowson (1976) calculated that if all the calcium required for six months of successful lactation were supplied from skeletal stores, the result would be a decrease of 6 percent in the skeleton's calcium content, an amount which may be too small to be detected with current methods of assessment.

Serum retinol levels seem low among several populations of lactating women, but it is not clear what role lactation plays in this phenomenon. However, Devadas et al. (1978) found an adequate mean retinol level among lactating Indian women, although intakes were inadequate.

Bates et al. (1981) examined riboflavin status in lactating women. They found a significantly higher erythrocyte glutathione reductase activity coefficient among lactating Gambian women as compared with healthy British controls, indicating deficient stores of riboflavin. Riboflavin intakes among Gambian women were also deficient.

Although the vitamin and mineral intakes of lactating women are often very low in comparison with recommendations, clinical and biochemical deficiency signs are not as prevalent. With low intakes, absorption and metabolization of vitamins and minerals may be enhanced (Whitehead, 1983) or the effects on maternal nutritional status of low intakes may be at the subclinical level. That most studies show that vitamin and mineral supplementation of lactating women brings about increases in the vitamin and mineral content of breast milk (Bates et al., 1983; Belavady, 1980; Coward et al., 1984) suggests that habitual low intakes may be compromising a lactating woman's ability to function optimally.

Anthropometric Measures

As with other indicators of nutritional status, there is no clear effect of lactation on maternal anthropometric measures. As table VII-5 illustrates, many studies have found that lactating women lose weight, but it is not clear whether the loss is only of stores laid down during pregnancy, or in excess of them. Only two studies, in Guatemala (Delgado et al., 1981;

and Valverde *et al.*, 1981), compared weight during lactation to an initial weight, although the baseline weights were measured during the first trimester or first half of pregnancy, when some slight weight change may have already occurred. Delgado *et al.* found that after 12 months of lactation, supplemented women had lost .90 kg. over their first trimester weights, while Valverde *et al.* found mean weight after 12 months of lactation did not fall below the mean weight in the first half of pregnancy.

In a study in the Gambia, Paul *et al.* (1979b) found lactating women lost weight only during the rainy season, a time of heavy agricultural labor and food shortages resulting in highly inadequate intakes. Even nonpregnant, nonlactating women lost weight during this season. At other times of the year, lactating women maintained their weight, or, if they continued to lactate after the rainy season, actually gained weight, even on low caloric intakes. Weight gains among lactating women after the rainy season occurred sooner than any increase in breast milk output, suggesting that maternal stores were being replenished at the expense of breast milk production.

A dietary intake below recommended levels can be compensated for by changes in metabolic demands for nutrients. A significant reduction in demand could result from a decrease in physical activity or production of a lower quantity of breast milk. Few studies have investigated these factors individually and none has considered how they might act together to alleviate the impact of a dietary intake well below recommended levels. Studies thus far have focused on calories and have not considered ways by which other nutrients might be conserved.

Physical Activity

Schutz *et al.* (1980) investigated energy intakes and expenditures of 18 lactating women and 6 nonpregnant, nonlactating controls in Guatemala. Excluding the energy cost of breast milk production, they found no significant difference in total daily energy expenditure of the two groups, nor in energy expenditure during different typical tasks.

In a detailed study of two villages in New Guinea, Norgan *et al.* (1974) found pregnant women in both had the same gross daily energy expenditures as their nonpregnant counterparts, although because of their increased weights, the pregnant women had lower energy expenditures per kg body mass. Norgan and colleagues reported no information on energy expenditure of lactating women. Durnin (1980) reported that in a subsequent study in one of the villages, energy expenditure was reduced in lactation, especially in the first six months and with the first child, but gave no figure. Total energy expenditure data were not given for pregnant and lactating women separately, but in one village, energy expenditure of all women was, on average, 400 kcal higher than their daily intake. There was, however, no evidence of weight loss.

McGuire (1979) studied the time allocation and energy expenditures of a small sample of lactating, pregnant and nonpregnant, nonlactating women in Guatemala. Statistical analyses were performed on differences between lactating and pregnant women but not between lactating and nonpregnant, nonlactating women. Broad categories of activities were evaluated based on time and energy costs. The mean daily energy expenditure of lactating women, (excluding the cost of breast milk production) measured by time/ motion studies and heart rate monitoring was significantly lower than that of pregnant women, and less than that of nonpregnant, nonlactating women. Lactating women used between 200 and 400 kcal per day less than pregnant women, depending on the method used to measure energy expenditure. On a body weight basis, however, energy expenditures were not significantly different.

Breast Milk Output

The impact of dietary intake on quantity and quality of breast milk is briefly reviewed in chapter 5.

Dietary recommendations for lactating women are based on a daily milk output of 850 ml/day with an energy content of 72 kcal/100 ml (WHO, 1973). Reviewing studies on the breast milk production of women in poorly nourished communities, Jelliffe and Jelliffe (1978b) concluded that an average of 500–700 ml. was produced daily in the first six months of lactation. Using the lower limit of 500 ml, with an energy content of 72 kcal/100 ml and conversion efficiency of 80 percent, approximately 315 calories (or 11 percent of the recommended intake) would be conserved by a reduction in breast milk output. This is a considerable savings, but does not come close to meeting the gap in calories (often in excess of 1,000 kcal/day) experienced by many Third World lactating women.

Maternal Depletion

It is commonly felt that, under conditions prevalent in developing countries, women undergoing repeated pregnancies and prolonged lactation experience a general deterioration of their health and nutritional status called the *maternal depletion syndrome* (D. B. Jelliffe, 1966; E. F. P. Jelliffe, 1976; Royston, 1982). Because of the long time span required to study such a phenomenon adequately, there are few good studies on the subject. Most have been cross-sectional and have not controlled for confounding variables, such as age.

E. F. Patrice Jelliffe (1976) mentioned that Chimbu women in New Guinea experience a weight decline with each reproductive cycle, although she gave no data and it is not clear whether age was controlled for. Kusin *et al.* (1979) found that the percentage of Javanese mothers with acceptable nutritional status decreased with parity (although age was not controlled for). In New Guinea, Harrison *et al.* (1975) found parity not significantly correlated with weight or ponderal index (height $\div \sqrt[3]{\text{weight}}$) but highly correlated to decline in several skinfold measures, even after controlling for age. Rowland and Paul (1981) found primiparous Gambian women could sustain lactation longer than multiparous women, suggesting that repeated reproductive cycles resulted in a deterioration of maternal nutritional health.

However, from the same studies in the Gambia on pregnant and lactating women, Prentice *et al.* (1981) found no change in body weight with parity and that women whose parity was below average for their age did not weigh more than average-parity women in the same age group. In a large cross-sectional study of women from various cultural settings in five countries, no consistent relationship was found between ponderal index and parity when age was controlled for (Omran and Standley, 1976). A relationship was observed only in Lebanon, and, in this case, ponderal index decreased with parity greater than four, indicating that higher parity women were heavier. In New Guinea, Norgan *et al.* (1974) found no change in body mass with repeated pregnancies; neither did Rajalakshmi (1971) among poor Indian women.

Omran and Standley (1976) studied the relationship between parity and iron status in five countries. In two, there was no relationship between parity and hemoglobin when age was controlled for. In Iran, hemoglobin decreased slightly with parity for women less than 30 years old. A decline with parity was also observed among Lebanese women between ages 30 and 39 and in Phillippine women older than 25. In a study on calcium status among high-parity Bantu women, Walker *et al.* (1972) found no radiological evidence of bone loss, even though calcium intake was low.

Apparently, maternal depletion may be a problem in some cultures and not in others. A lifelong deterioration in maternal health may be influenced by a broad range of social and economic factors such as unsanitary living conditions for low-income families, and lack of adequate health care services. In studies where maternal depletion has been found to be associated with parity, it is not clear what role lactation plays independent of the effects of repeated pregnancies.

CONCLUSIONS

The differential effects of infant-feeding methods on women's nutritional status have not been adequately studied. Effects of breast-feeding specifically have been examined to some extent, but results are not consistent, and methodological problems preclude drawing conclusions. Dietary intakes of nonpregnant, nonlactating women in developing countries are often inadequate when compared with current standards (Hamilton *et al.*, 1984). From current data, it appears that lactating women do not significantly increase their dietary intake over that of their nonpregnant, nonlactating state. Their diets are consequently often even more inadequate, when compared with recommendations, than those of their nonpregnant, nonlactating counterparts. This apparently inadequate intake may result from data collection methodologies which consistently underestimate actual intakes or may be because recommendations are considerably higher than actual individual requirements. Or the dietary intakes of lactating women may indeed be inadequate.

Whether and to what degree these apparently inadequate intakes affect the ability of lactating women to function is not clear. Anthropometric and biochemical data show some adverse effects of lactation, but not to the extent expected from the magnitude of the supposed dietary deficiencies. The impact on physical activity and breast milk production has not been studied carefully enough to draw conclusions. Unfortunately, information on the impact of lactation on different nutritional status indicators comes from studies on different populations. No one study has looked at all the major factors influencing nutritional status to explain the apparent inconsistency between dietary data and other more functional measures of the nutritional status of lactating women.

Other important issues regarding the impact of infant feeding on the mother's nutritional health have not been adequately investigated. No study has examined the impact of feeding other infant foods on the nutritional status of a nonlactating, postpartum woman. Whether a longer duration of breast-feeding has a more pronounced effect is also not clear, nor whether the effect, if any, of infant feeding on maternal nutritional status operates through a *dose-response mechanism* or a *threshold mechanism*. In a mixed-feeding situation, does maternal nutritional status vary continuously with the proportion of breast milk or other foods fed to the infant, or is maternal nutritional status constant until some threshold level in use of breast milk or other foods is reached? Resolution of these issues is needed for the formulation of recommendations on infant feeding. These issues await careful research.

8
INFANT FEEDING, FECUNDITY, AND FERTILITY

In this chapter we examine the influence of infant-feeding practices on fecundity and fertility. For purposes of this review, breast-feeding is considered to be different from other types of infant feedings in its fertility-suppressing effect. In this framework, no direct role in fertility suppression is attributable to other types of infant feeding. For example, if other foods or milks are being substituted for the nutrients provided by breast milk, breast suckling may significantly decline resulting in a series of hormonal events leading to the postpartum resumption of fecundity. The choice of other foods or milks may result in a decline in maternal nutritional status by channeling limited household food monies towards preferential purchases of infant foods. The deterioration in maternal nutritional status may then result in lengthening postpartum infecundity. We examine the various pathways by which breast-feeding can influence fecundity and fertility.

Several terms should be defined. *Fertility* means "actual reproductive performance—whether applied to an individual or group" (IUSSP, 1958:38). *Fecundity* refers to "the capacity of a man, a woman or a couple to participate in reproduction, (i.e., the production of a live child)" (IUSSP, 1958:38). *Infecundity, sterility,* or *physiological infertility* are terms referring to lack of this capacity for conception in a menstrual cycle (IUSSP, 1958:41). *Amenorrhea* denotes the absence of menstruation and *anovulation,* the absence of ovulation. The term *lactational amenorrhea* describes the delay in postpartum return of menstruation that is extended in lactating women.

THEORETICAL PATHWAYS

In figure VIII-1, infant feeding is postulated to influence fertility and fecundity through several pathways. Infant feeding may affect maternal hormonal levels through suckling or through influencing use of hormonal

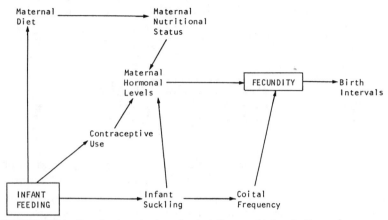

FIGURE VIII-1   Postulated mechanisms for the influence of infant feeding on postpartum fecundity and fertility.

contraceptive agents which in turn alter fecundity and thereby affect fertility. Infant feeding may modify maternal nutritional status through the nutrient cost of breast milk production or through influencing the mother's dietary intakes, which may directly change her hormonal levels, as well as indirectly by affecting infant suckling. Finally, infant feeding may alter coital behavior and thereby affect fertility.

Infant Feeding and Maternal Hormonal Levels

Postpartum maternal hormonal levels, crucial to the return of fecundity, can be signficantly influenced by the suckling associated with breast-feeding. In fact, some consider the suckling stimulus (resulting in elevated serum prolactin levels) to be the major determinant of the prolonged anovulation of lactation (Habicht et al., 1985). Other types of infant feeding (less or no breast-feeding) could influence fecundity by diminishing or excluding suckling, thereby reducing the stimulus for hormonal suppression of fecundity.

Use of hormonal contraceptives obviously can influence maternal hormone levels and delay the return of fecundity. A breast-feeding mother may believe she is fully protected through lactation alone and choose not to use a hormonal contraceptive (e.g., Millman, 1985). Another mother may choose to use a hormonal contraceptive believing that she will not significantly diminish her milk production or endanger her infant while using these pills and would be fully confident of being protected against pregnancy.

Current evidence indicates that lactation directly affects fecundity through neurohormonal mechanisms triggered by infant suckling which prolong the delay in return of ovulation (Delvoye *et al.*, 1976; Short, 1982; Tucker, 1979; Tyson, 1976). Pituitary hormone prolactin (PRL) is key in this process. Circulating concentrations of PRL and duration of postpartum infecundity are highly correlated (Bonnar *et al.*, 1975; Delvoye *et al.*, 1977; Howie and McNeilly, 1982). Higher PRL levels are found as a result of lactation behaviors associated with longer duration of postpartum amenorrhea such as full compared to partial breast-feeding (B. A. Gross and Eastman, 1979; McNeilly *et al.*, 1980; Tyson *et al.*, 1976), higher breast-feeding frequency (Delvoye *et al.*, 1977; Noel *et al.*, 1974), greater suckling intensity (Aono *et al.*, 1977; Tyson *et al.*, 1978); and longer continuation of night feedings (Howie *et al.*, 1982a,b). When breast-feeding is totally discontinued, prolactin levels drop precipitously with a concomitant rise in luteinizing hormones (LH) and estradiol, indicating a return of ovarian activity with ovulation occurring within 14–30 days thereafter (McNeilly *et al.*, 1981). Nipple stimulation appears to induce prolactin release. When the nipple is anesthetized or totally denervated as a result of reduction mammoplasty, PRL is not released in response to suckling (Tyson, 1977). Nipple stimulation alone without lactation can result in elevated PRL levels (McNeilly, 1977).

Several researchers suggest physiological mechanisms by which PRL might suppress ovarian cycles, thus postponing the return of postpartum fecundity in lactating women. Habicht *et al.* (1985) suggest that in the early postpartum period prolactin may act directly on the ovaries to inhibit its response to the gonadotropins, LH, and follicle-stimulating hormone (FSH). PRL may directly inhibit ovarian steroidogenesis (McNatty *et al.*, 1974), inhibit the secretion of gonadotropin-releasing-hormone (GnRH) (Baird *et al.*, 1979), impair pituitary responsiveness to GnRH (London *et al.*, 1977), or hypothalamic sensitivity to estrogen (Habicht *et al.*, 1985). The episodic release and surge of LH required for ovulation would be prevented by this effect on the hypothalamus. Failure of ovarian follicular development and lactational amenorrhea may result from suckling-induced high PRL levels which suppress LH (Glasier *et al.*, 1983) but not FSH postpartum. Ovulations occurring prior to weaning are usually "infertile," with a deficient corpus luteum (B. A. Gross and Eastman, 1983b; McNeilly et al., 1981). This insufficiency has been noted in several studies as an additional effect of lactation on ovarian cycles (Delvoye et al., 1980; Duchen and McNeilly, 1980; Howie et al., 1981; Jain et al., 1979).

Recent evidence suggests that prolactin may not be the only pathway through which suckling influences postpartum infecundity. In a study involving rhesus monkeys, prolactin secretion was inhibited with bromocriptine but suckling suppressed gonadotropin secretion and sustained amenorrhea still occurred (Schallenberger et al., 1981). While suckling may influence fertility through prolactin-dependent as well as prolactin-independent pathways (Short, 1983), the unravelling of these mechanisms is needed.

The mechanisms responsible for lactational suppression of postpartum fecundity are complex, involving factors other than prolactin alone. They include neural response to suckling, suppression of LH secretion, and various target organs including the hypothalamus and ovaries. An integrated system for these factors is yet to be elucidated (McNeilly et al., 1981). No one really knows the precise mechanisms by which infant suckling by itself and through its effects on prolactin levels influences gonadotropins to bring about the suppression of "fertile" ovulation. We do know that lactation through infant suckling affects maternal hormonal levels which are intimately linked with the return of postpartum ovulation.

Infant Feeding and Maternal Nutritional Status

An infant-feeding method that affects maternal diet and nutritional status (see Chapter 7) may in turn affect fecundity through several distinct means. A mother's nutritional status or diet may affect her hormonal levels indirectly through infant suckling. Studies suggest maternal nutritional status or diet can influence lactation performance characteristics including quantity and quality of breast milk (see Chapter 5). Poor maternal nutritional status or diet may lead to declines in breast milk quantity and quality and to earlier supplementation of the infant with other milks or foods, which reduces suckling or causes earlier cessation of lactation. On the other hand, an unsupplemented infant may suckle with more vigor, eliciting a greater maternal prolactin response and extending the length of postpartum infecundity.

A mother's nutritional status or diet may affect her hormonal levels directly. Nutritional status influences individual growth and development and female endocrine status (Brasel, 1978). In populations where chronic undernutrition is common, women also may be subfecund (Frisch, 1975, 1978; Mosley, 1979). Although the hypothesis is still under dispute (Billewicz *et al.*, 1976; Cameron, 1976; F. E. Johnston *et al.*, 1975; Reeves, 1979), Frisch has tried to document a body fat threshold for ovulation. Essentially, Frisch and her colleagues argue that a critically low percentage of body fat is a determinant delaying onset of menses. They estimate that 22 percent of body weight as fat is needed to maintain normal menstrual function. If malnourished women are subfecund or have longer periods of postpartum amenorrhea, infecundity in lactating women may be a separate and additional function of their nutritional status. We review evidence of the effect of maternal nutritional status on fecundity later in this chapter.

Infant Feeding and Coital Frequency

Breast-feeding may influence coital behavior. Some cultures prohibit sexual intercourse for the duration of breast-feeding (Liskin, 1981). In many regions of the world, this leads to one or two years of postpartum abstinence and represents a major source of couple-months of protection against fertility. Liskin reports recent declines in the practice of postpartum abstinence, however. In some cultures, women sleep with the baby they are breast-feeding, which may also inhibit sexual contact. Other researchers (N. A. Newton, 1973) report an increased interest in intercourse among women who are breast-feeding. The possibility of selection bias has been raised in considering the latter circumstance. More sexually expressive women may also be more likely to breast-feed (Anderson, 1983). Night-feedings and fatigue associated with breast-feeding may alter frequency of coitus, as might postpartum depression (Adler and Cox, 1983), reported to occur more frequently in fully breast-feeding women. Fertility may be affected by any of these factors, which would result in a decline in coital frequency.

METHODOLOGICAL ISSUES

Outcome Variables: Fecundity and Fertility

Because fecundity is not exhibited through readily discernible signs and symptoms, the precise determination of its return postpartum must be measured through clinical and biochemical tests which determine whether ovulation has resumed and whether the hormonal environment associated with fecundity has been restored. Tests of vaginal cytology, hormonal assays, basal temperature charts, and cervical mucus records can be helpful for this purpose, but have rarely been used in epidemiological research on this topic because of the expense of the procedures and the careful and consistent cooperation needed from study participants.

Since ovulation and other clinical aspects of fecundity have not been easily measurable in the past, related measurements have been reported as proxies, including return of menstruation postpartum and serum prolactin levels. Postpartum return of menstruation, although not synonymous with ovulation or fecundity, is a readily identifiable characteristic considered an indicator of the other conditions. Robert G. Potter *et al.* (1979) estimated that approximately 70 percent of women who have resumed menstruating postpartum will also be ovulatory. Correlation coefficients between anovulation and postpartum amenorrhea are also consistently high (Menken *et al.*, 1981; Pérez, 1979). None of these facts, however, provides assurance that amenorrheic women are actually infecund, since ovulation may resume before return of the menses. An estimated 2 to 10 percent of lactating women in developing countries conceive during the period of lactational amenorrhea (Badraoui and Hefnawi, 1979; Simpson-Hebert and Huffman, 1981).

All ovulations are not "fertile" and the hormonal environment supportive of conception must also be in place for fecundity to be present. Researchers often determine serum prolactin levels because of their linkage with return of postpartum fecundity. Unlike hormonal assays for ovulation which require serial measurements of several gonadotropic hormones and 24-hour urine collections, serum prolactin levels are usually measured at a single time and reported as "basal" or "postsuckling" levels. However, serum prolactin levels are subject to diurnal variation with nighttime peaks that differ depending on the length of time postpartum (Tyson *et al.*, 1978), the interval between breast-feedings, the duration of the breast-feeding, the intensity of suckling during the feeding, and the time during or after feeding when the serum sample is drawn (Aono *et al.*, 1977). Basal prolactin levels in women whose infants nurse frequently may be higher because of the shortened time between suckling episodes. If night-feedings are eliminated, a significant decline appears in basal PRL, attributed to the long period of PRL decline each night. Additional, but, controversial influences may include maternal stress (Noel *et al.*, 1972) and fat intake (Hill and Wynder, 1976). Although significantly higher basal levels of serum prolactin are associated with longer durations of postpartum amenorrhea, a precise threshold for a fecundity-suppressing level is yet to be established.

Fertility is often reported in terms of *birth intervals*—"the intervals between successive births" (IUSSP, 1958:37). Longer birth intervals are indicative of longer periods of postpartum infecundity in populations not using contraceptive methods. Use of this measure, however, should consider nonproductive pregnancies (miscarriages, spontaneous abortions, stillbirths) which may have occurred during the birth interval.

Exposure Variable: Breast-feeding

Breast-feeding classifications applied variably to study participants have caused problems. This issue has been carefully reviewed in chapter 2 and by Notzon (1984) and Habicht *et al.* (1985). In studies of breast-feeding, fecundity, and fertility, various lactation performance characteristics have been used as independent variables with differences noted in fecundity and fertility. These characteristics include full versus partial breast-feeding. All of these characteristics can be related to infant suckling behavior (see figure VIII-2). Suckling appears to influence maternal hormonal levels and thereby fecundity directly. The other lactation characteristics can be considered aspects of suckling, but there are questions about their measurement.

Evidence points to differences in length of postpartum amenorrhea between women who fully and partially breast-feed; the question of how supplementation affects suckling behavior has not been established. It is not clear in these studies whether supplementary food was given before or after a breast-feeding or in lieu of it. Suggested mechanisms for the influence of supplementation on suckling behavior include an appetite- and suckling-blunting effect. Some evidence exists for the appetite-blunting effect of supplementation. Huffman (1985) noted in her Bangladeshi population that feeding solid supplements to infants was more likely to be associated with

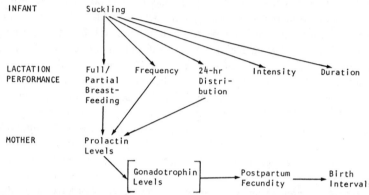

FIGURE VIII-2   Relationships among lactation performance characteristics and their effects on fecundity and fertility.

shortened periods of postpartum amenorrhea for the mother than feeding liquid supplements. A suckling-blunting effect of supplementation may operate in those infants taking supplements through nippled bottles.

There are also measurement problems with the variables *lactation frequency* and *intensity of suckling*. Neither has a rigorous definition. Studies which report lactation frequency as a variable do not state whether differentiation is made between nutritive and nonnutritive suckling at the breast and whether differences in suckling result in different hormonal responses. Aono *et al.* (1977) noted increased prolactin levels with constant breast pump stimulation for an average nursing period. This finding suggests that more suckling as such might induce higher prolactin levels and thereby delay postpartum fecundity. It is further unclear whether frequency of lactation refers to the number of times the infant was put to the breast or to the number of suckling episodes of whatever duration or type. An infant might suck the breast more than once during a period in which it was put to the breast. The researcher may ask for frequencies of feeds during a particular period of time which would include partial feeds or omit a feed that occurred just after the conclusion of the timed period (Habicht, *et al.*, 1985). In some cultures mothers carry their infants in a way that facilitates "demand" feeding (Gussler and Breisemeister, 1980). By wearing clothing with a loose bodice and fastening the baby in a carrying sling in front of her bosom, the mother can easily respond to the infant's cry for feeding. Accuracy of recall of breast-feeding frequency in these situations has been questioned (Zeitlin *et al.*, 1980).

Intensity of suckling, while critical in inducing hormonal suppression of fecundity, is an entity largely undefined and unmeasured. Some studies have relied on the mother's subjective judgment of the degree of intensity of each suckling episode (B. A. Gross and Eastman, 1983b). The majority of studies identifying intensity of suckling as an important factor have only provided a vague description for this variable.

Habicht *et al.* (1985) have noted that analysis should only include breast-feeding duration preceding the return of the outcome variable of interest— menstruation, ovulation, or "fertile" ovulation (fecundity) and not the total breast-feeding period. This point is important since only that portion of breast-feeding which could potentially influence the particular outcome should properly be considered in any analysis. Also, instead of aggregating breast-feeding practice into a single variable, Habicht and colleagues sum it into all relevant portions which includes a full and a partial breast-feeding effect. Habicht *et al.* show in their analysis of Malaysian data that more stable estimates of the breast-feeding effect on fecundity are possible using this more precise analysis of breast-feeding. Similarly, other dimensions of lactation performance which affect neurohormonal response should be considered. See figure VIII-2.

Confounding Variables

Oral contraceptives

A mother's use of contraceptives in the presence of any type of infant feeding obviously confounds the effect of feeding on fecundity and fertility. Lactating women using contraceptives are different from other lactating women since they are "infecund" by virtue of their contraceptives. Some oral contraceptives appear to have a lactation-suppressing effect. Estrogen-containing contraceptives or those with an estrogenic effect may significantly reduce milk yields (Hull, 1981; Laukaran, 1981) in some cases (McCann *et al.*, 1981). Combination-type oral contraceptives with as little as 30μg of estrogen have reduced milk volume by as much as 40 percent within three to six weeks of use, and their early postpartum use was associated in a dose-related manner with shortening breast-feeding duration (WHO/NRC, 1983). Progestin-only contraceptives appear to have no effect on milk yields or may increase them (McCann *et al.*, 1981) and are associated with a significant but small decrease in total breast milk fat (WHO/NRC, 1983). Progestogen-only and nonhormonal methods have little or no effect on duration of breast-feeding while injectable contraceptives have been associated with increased duration (WHO/NRC, 1983).

Lactating oral contraceptive users who note a reduction in milk yields may opt to supplement their infants with other milks or foods or stop breast-feeding altogether. Thus lactating oral contraceptive users are likely to have different lactation performance characteristics than nonusers as well as being infecund.

Maternal age and smoking

Others have noted a difference in breast-feeding and fecundity related to maternal age (Jain *et al.*, 1979) but have determined that differences could be attributed to differences in breast-feeding performance characteristics associated with age rather than age itself. Habicht *et al.* (forthcoming) noted in Malaysia that physiological as well as behavioral differences may have accounted for lengthening the duration of postpartum anovulation from age 20 upwards. Although the data suggest a behavioral difference relating to cohort membership even in the case of partial breast-feeding, multicollinearity in the data did not allow for sorting separately effects of physiological and behavioral differences with age. It is not clear to what extent such data problems existed in studies which reported more definitive findings and whether the analytic methods used sufficiently corrected for those problems. Further work is needed to clarify whether maternal age has an independent and, therefore, confounding effect on the breast-feeding and fecundity relationship.

Following up on the lead of animal studies which showed an inhibition of PRL response to lactation with nicotine, Andersen and Schiøler (1982) examined the relationship of smoking to PRL levels in nursing mothers. In general, women who smoked had shorter periods of breast-feeding and those who smoked more than 15 cigarettes a day had lower basal levels of PRL early in the puerperium. This finding suggests that smoking may hasten the return of fecundity by reducing PRL levels. It may be possible to test this hypothesis in developing countries of Southeast Asia where some rural women traditionally use tobacco and are also likely to breast-feed for a long duration.

REVIEW OF STUDIES

Although most women are physiologically incapable of conceiving (infecund) for at least four to six weeks after delivery (Sharman, 1951), longer periods of natural infecundity, as much as two or more years, have been observed in lactating women. The traditional practice of long breast-feeding and its associated lactational amenorrhea of one to two years or more still occurs in some developing countries (DaVanzo and Haaga, 1982; WHO/NRC, 1983).

Breast-Feeding Practice and Fecundity/Fertility

Table VIII-1 summarizes some of the studies which examine the hypothesis that breast-feeding is associated with a longer period of postpartum infecundity and thereby infertility. McCann *et al.* (1981) give a more comprehensive review. The consensus of these studies is that breast-feeding is associated with longer periods of postpartum amenorrhea compared to that occurring in nonbreast-feeders. Full breast-feeding is associated with a longer period of postpartum amenorrhea than partial breast-feeding. Differences in measured return of ovulation (Pérez *et al.*, 1972) and birth intervals (Jain *et al.*, 1979) have also been noted with breast-feeders experiencing a longer delay in return of ovulation postpartum and having longer intervals between births.

A Taiwanese study (Jain *et al.*, 1979) indicates a possible separate effect of lactation on fecundity aside from suppression of menstruation. This finding is also suggested in Chile (Perez *et al.*, 1972) where differences in ovulation indicated that lactation may also influence whether the first postpartum menstrual cycles are ovulatory. Others have made similar findings (Delvoye *et al.*, 1980). There are also indications of subfecundity, for example inadequate luteal function, even with the return of menstruation among lactating women (Berman *et al.*, 1972; Howie and McNeilly, 1982; Pérez *et al.*, 1972; Simpson-Hebert, 1977). Howie *et al.* (1982a) not only found that return of ovulation was postponed significantly longer in lactating mothers than in bottle-feeders but also that normal cycling did not return until their babies were weaned completely.

Infant suckling has been implicated as the key fecundity-suppressing effect of lactation. More frequent (Delvoye *et al.*, 1977; Howie *et al.*,

TABLE VIII-1

Studies supporting the hypothesis: Breast-feeding is associated with longer postpartum infecundity and infertility

Study	Study Date & Site	N	Feeding Groups	Outcome Variable	Outcome Measure	Control Variables	Findings
COHORT							
Malkani & Mirchandani, 1960[1]	Aug. 1957–June 1958 New Delhi	452	BFs, NBFs, postabortion patients	PA	RMR	None	NBF: $\bar{X}$ PA = 58 days; BF: $\bar{X}$ PA = 5.25 mos
RETROSPECTIVE							
Osteria, 1973	May 1973 Laguna, Philippines	180	BFs, NBFs	PA	RMR	Oral CU	NBF: $\bar{X}$ PA = 1.9 mos; BF: $\bar{X}$ PA = 9.8 mos
Crisol & Phillips, 1975	1974, Philippines	2365[a]	BFs, NBFs	PA	RMR	NBFs	NBF: $\bar{X}$ PA = 3.4 mos; BF: $\bar{X}$ PA = 9.2 mos
Singarimbun & Manning, 1976	Apr. 1969–Mar. 1970 Indonesia	772	BFs; child died/stillborn	PA; BIs	RM BIs	Abstinence duration	

TABLE VIII-1 (continued)

Study	Study Date & Site	N	Feeding Groups	Outcome Variable	Outcome Measure	Control Variables	Findings
Jain et al., 1979	1967 Taiwan	5000	BFs, NBFs	PA length, BI length	RMR, BI	CU	NBF: $\overline{X}$ PA = 4.4 mos + 0.4 mos @ mos of BF NBF: $\overline{X}$ B1 = 24.8 mos BF: $\overline{X}$ B1 = 24.8 mos + 0.7 mos @ mos of BF + 0.4 mos @ mos of PA
PROSPECTIVE							
Berman et al., 1972	1966–70 Alaska, USA	299	BFs, NBFs	PA; pregnancy	Menstrual diaries (nurse follow-up)	CU; Eskimo	NBF: PA approx. 2 mos BF: $\overline{X}$ PA 10 mos estimated ovulations NBF: 3 mos P BF: 4 mos P

TABLE VIII-1 (continued)

Study	Study Date & Site	N	Feeding Groups	Outcome Variable	Outcome Measure	Control Variables	Findings
Perez et al., 1972	1965–68 Chile	281	BFs (full & partial), NBFs	PA; ovulation	Weekly clinic follow-up; daily BBT charting; vaginal wall smears; cervical mucus study; endometrial biopsy	SES, rhythm use	NBF: $\overline{X}$ PA = 1.5 mos; BF: < 17.5 mos PA > 1 yr ovulation; NBF: $\overline{X}$ 49 days P (SD 12 days); BF: $\overline{X}$ 112 days P (SD 71 days)
Osteria, 1978	1973–75 Manila	794	BFs (full & partial), NBFs	PA length	Monthly follow-up of MR, pregnancy	None	NBF: $\overline{X}$ PA = 1 mo; Partial BF = 3 mos; Full BF = 9 mos
LONGITUDINAL							
Howie et al., 1982b[2]	n.d. Scotland	35	BFs, NBFs	—	MR, ovulation	None	NBF: $\overline{X}$ PA = 8.1 wks $\overline{X}$ PAn = 10.8 wks; BF: $\overline{X}$ PA = 32.5 wks $\overline{X}$ PAn = 36.4 wks

Notes: BBT = basal body temperature; BFs = breast-feeding mothers; BI = birth interval; CU = contraceptive use; MR = menstrual resumption; NBFs = nonbreast-feeding mothers; P = postpartum; PA = postpartum amenorrhea; PAn = postpartum anovulation; RMR = reported resumption of menstruation; SD = standard deviation; SES = socioeconomic status; $\overline{X}$ = mean.
The breast-feeding measure here is (1) duration and full vs partial; (2) here, numbering and timing of suckling episodes, full/partial; in all other studies in this table, the measure is duration alone.
[a]Weighted

1982a; Noel *et al.*, 1974) and more intense suckling (Aono *et al.*, 1977; Howie *et al.*, 1982a; Tyson *et al.*, 1978) are associated with higher prolactin levels and longer durations of lactational amenorrhea. Maintenance of night-feeds and its consequent shortening of the most likely longest interval between suckling episodes (B. A. Gross and Eastman, 1983b) has been suggested as the most important factor influencing the mean interval length between suckling sessions and thereby maternal prolactin levels (Howie and McNeilly, 1982; Wood, forthcoming).

Indirect evidence for this suckling effect is based on studies examining partial versus full breast-feeding and fecundity. A reduction in suckling is expected with partial breast-feeding. Women who were fully breast-feeding have had significantly higher prolactin levels (Lunn *et al.*, 1980) and longer durations of lactational amenorrhea compared to lactating women who were supplementing their infant with other foods (Chen *et al.*, 1979; McNeilly *et al.*, 1980; Pérez *et al.*, 1972).

Providing supplementary foods is associated with changes in lactation performance characteristics—suckling duration (Andersen and Schiøler, 1982; Howie *et al.*, 1982a), frequency (Howie *et al.*, 1982a), and 24-hour distribution (Andersen and Schiøler, 1982). One study noted, however, that suckling intensity was not affected by supplementation (Andersen and Schiøler, 1982). Timing of the introduction of supplements also appears to affect serum PRL levels importantly. PRL levels peak just after delivery and start to decline thereafter. The earlier supplements are introduced into the infant's diet, the greater the subsequent decline in prolactin (B. A. Gross and Eastman, 1983a). The rate of increase of supplementary foods (Howie *et al.*, 1982a), especially solid supplements (B. A. Gross and Eastman, 1983a), appears to shorten postpartum infecundity.

Unsupplemented lactation even as long as one year or more (Prema and Ravindranath, 1982) has not been shown to postpone return of the menses indefinitely. Rather there appears to be a time-dependent decay in PRL levels following delivery to a threshold postpartum level seen in normal, nonpregnant, nonlactating women (Habicht *et al.*, 1985). Once this threshold is reached, normal cycling and ovulation are reestablished.

Several reports attempt to quantify the breast-feeding and postpartum infecundity relationship in relation to overall demographic effect, couple-years of protection, and length of postponed fecundity. Breast-feeding has been touted as a major determinant of fertility levels in populations not using modern contraceptive techniques (Short, 1983). Breast-feeding provides an estimated 31×10^6 couple-years of protection as compared to 24

$\times 10^6$ for artificial contraceptives used over one year, assuming eight months of lactational infecundity for rural mothers and four for urban mothers (Rosa, 1975). The net demographic consequences of lactational infecundity are difficult to sort out since lower infant mortality is also associated with breast-feeding (Knodel, 1977).

The specification of breast-feeding characteristics associated with fertility suppression has also been attempted. McNeilly *et al.* (1983) estimate that at least five suckling episodes more than ten minutes in length (65 minutes minimum daily) are needed to suppress fertility. For those partially breast-feeding, a daily threshold ratio of breast-feeding episodes to supplementations of 4.5 to one was found to sustain both high PRL levels and anovulation (Andersen and Schiøler, 1982).

Various estimates of the length of postponed fecundity with breast-feeding average an extension of approximately 0.4 to 0.6 months of infecundity for every extra month of breast-feeding (Corsini, 1979; B. A. Gross, 1981; Jain *et al.*, 1979; Leridon, 1977), with a maximum of 40 months of postpartum infecundity (Potter and Kobrin, 1981). A recent estimate based on analyses of World Fertility Survey data (Goldman *et al.*, 1985) found an increase in waiting time to conception of three-fourths the duration of lactation plus 6.8 months. Data on the Papua New Guinean Gainj showed a median of approximately seven months between resumption of ovulation and next fertile conception (Wood *et al.*, forthcoming). Habicht *et al.* (1985) found a larger effect of breast-feeding—even partial breast-feeding—in their analysis of Malaysian data. They noted that a month of full breast-feeding resulted on average in more than one month of anovulation and that even partial breast-feeding strongly influenced postponement of fecundity.

Such estimates are of limited usefulness because of lack of consensus. Research continues to underscore the wide variations among lactating populations and individuals with similar durations of breast-feeding regarding the length of postpartum infecundity (Knodel, 1977; McCann *et al.*, 1981). Although lactation duration can affect duration of amenorrhea, we also know that the mother will eventually regain her fecundity. As the physiological and behavioral framework underlying the breast-feeding and postpartum infecundity relationship are more clearly delineated, better quantitative estimates will be possible.

Maternal Nutritional Status and Diet

Studies have reported longer duration of postpartum amenorrhea among lactating women who were poor, most of whom were chronically undernourished (Chávez and Martínez, 1973; Delgado *et al.*, 1978; Saxton and Serwadda, 1969). Table VIII-2 summarizes some research on maternal nutritional status and diet (independent of lactational effects) on fecundity.

Some studies indicated that maternal undernutrition leads to a delayed return of menstruation postpartum (Chen *et al.*, 1974; Saxton and Serwadda, 1969). Confounding variables in the early nutrition and fertility studies—differences in breast-feeding practices, socioeconomic status (Saxton and Serwadda, 1969), and seasonality (Chen *et al.*, 1974)—undermine the credibility of their nutrition and fecundity findings. Conflicting evidence showed that poorly nourished women had no significant weight loss during lactation (Belavady and Gopalan, 1959; Thomson *et al.*, 1966). No correlation was found between weight gain and timing of conception (Bongaarts and Delgado, 1979; Howell, 1979). More recent studies have found increased PRL levels among poorly nourished lactating women (Lunn *et al.*, 1980), and no differences in PRL among low-income Indian women when nutritional status is measured by weight for height (Shatrugna *et al.*, 1982).

Studies examining the effect of supplementing the diets of lactating, undernourished mothers are also cited as evidence for the link between nutrition and duration of lactational amenorrhea (Chávez and Martínez, 1973; Delgado *et al.*, 1978). This linkage can be criticized since important variables such as infant supplementation, which could have significantly shortened lactational amenorrhea by itself, were not considered. Recent studies in Bangladesh (Chowdhury, 1978; Huffman *et al.*, 1978, 1980) and reexaminations of Guatemalan data (Delgado *et al.*, 1978) could not find support for the Frisch hypothesis, for a significant impact of nutritional status of lactating women on length of postpartum amenorrhea, or on overall fertility rates. One study in India (Prema *et al.*, 1980), controlled for known confounding variables, found support for a separate maternal nutrition effect on postpartum amenorrhea. These findings need to be verified in other populations since in the Prema study earlier infant supplementation was associated with greater maternal weight, the maternal nutritional status variable used in that study.

TABLE VIII-2

Studies related to the hypothesis: Maternal nutritional status and diet have an independent and additive effect aside from effects on fertility

Study	Study Date & Site	N	Nutritional Status/Diet Measure	Lactation Measure	Outcome Variable	Outcome Measure	Supports Hypothesis	Control Variables	Findings
CROSS-SECTIONAL									
Prema et al., 1980	India	2250	Maternal	BF, NBF	PA length, inter-pregnancy interval	RMR, reported pregnancy history	[Higher wt associated with earlier supple-mentation]	SES, infant supplemen-tation (?), age, parity, lactation duration, contraceptive use	Higher body wt (> 55 kg) associated with shorter lac-tation dura-tion; higher body wt with same lactation duration associated with shorter PA
CROSS-SECTIONAL & RETROSPECTIVE DATA									
Caräel, 1978	1974–75 Zaire	749	Prior area nutrition survey results	Duration, full/ partial	PA length	RMR	?	Ecological areas; coital frequency not controlled	

TABLE VIII-2 (continued)

Study	Study Date & Site	N	Nutritional Status/Diet Measure	Lactation Measure	Outcome Variable	Outcome Measure	Supports Hypothesis	Control Variables	Findings
PROSPECTIVE									
Chávez & Martinez, 1973	1968–71 Mexico	64	Only for supplemented mothers: wt gain during pregnancy; hemoglobin levels	All lactating otherwise undifferentiated	Fecundity	Fertility recovery time (new pregnancy or RM)	?	SES, infant supplementation not controlled	Fertility recovery time: Unsupplemented = mean 14.0 ± 4 mos supplemented = mean 7.5 ± 2.6 mos
Chen et al., 1974	1969–71 Bangladesh	193	Not measured	Partial vs full BF	Fecundity	Reported LA duration; monthly pregnancy urine tests	?	Religion, contraceptive use, husband's absences, seasonal variation in RM & ovulation	Median PA length Nonlactating = 2 mos Lactating = 17 mos
Chowdhury, 1978	Nov. 1975– Nov. 1976	2218	Maternal ht, wt, arm circumference, hematocrit	Not stated	PA length	RMR	?	Length of husband's absences; lactation effect?	Nutritional status not significantly associated

TABLE VIII-2

Study	Study Date & Site	N	Nutritional Status/Diet Measure	Lactation Measure	Outcome Variable	Outcome Measure	Supports Hypothesis	Control Variables	Findings
PROSPECTIVE (continued)									
Delgado et al., 1978	1969–75 Guatemala	398	*Prenatal* Maternal home dietary intake, supplement consumption *Postnatal* Maternal anthropometry	Duration	PA length	@14 days menstruation & lactation monitoring	?	SES, infant supplementation not controlled	Better pregnancy nutritional status associated with longer PA
Huffman et al., 1978	1975 Matlab, Bangladesh	2048	Maternal ht & wt	BFs	PA length	RMR	No	Breast-feeders only	Nutritional status not significantly associated
Huffman et al., 1980	1975–76 Matlab, Bangladesh	171	Maternal ht & wt	BFF	PA length	RMR	No	Breast-feeders only	Slight effect of nutritional status on BI estimated to result in < 1 birth over women's reproductive span

TABLE VIII-2 (continued)

Study	Study Date & Site	N	Nutritional Status/Diet Measure	Lactation Measure	Outcome Variable	Outcome Measure	Supports Hypothesis	Control Variables	Findings
PROSPECTIVE (continued)									
Lunn et al., 1980	UK & Gambia 1979–80	30 119	Subsample: weighed food intake for home intake & supplement	Breast milk output by test-weighing, frequency	Plasma prolactin levels	Measured by double antibody radioimmunoassay	Yes	Breast-feeders only, SES	Significant reduction in prolactin levels with improved maternal diet
Lunn et al., 1981	1979–80 Gambia	119	Subsample: weighed food intake for home intake & supplement	Breast milk output by test-weighing, frequency	Conceptions by plasma estradiol, PA length by plasma progesterone	Measured by radioimmunoassay	Yes	Breast-feeders only, SES	Plasma estradiol & progesterone concentration indication indicating RM & return of ovulation occurring significantly earlier in supplemented women; LA shortened by 6 mos in supplemented lactating women

TABLE VIII-2 (continued)

Study	Study Date & Site	N	Nutritional Status/Diet Measure	Lactation Measure	Outcome Variable	Outcome Measure	Supports Hypothesis	Control Variables	Findings
UNSTATED DESIGN	nd								
Saxton & Serwadda 1969	Rwanda Uganda Rwanda Tanzania	259 210 186 148	Not stated	Not stated	Fecundity, fertility	RM, BI	?	Differences in BF practices not controlled	PA longer, among "well-nourished" Ugandans vs marginally nourished Rwandans

Notes: BF = breast-feeding; BFF = breast-feeding frequency; BI = birth interval; LA = lactational amenorrhea; nd = no date; PA = postpartum amenorrhea; RM = resumption of menstruation; RMR = reported menstrual resumption; SES = socioeconomic status

The Gambian studies (Lunn *et al.*, 1980, 1981) have provided the most substantial evidence to date for the influence of maternal nutritional status and diet on postpartum infecundity. In these studies, careful measurements of maternal diet, anthropometry, milk yields, and hormonal levels were made over an 18-month period in 119 lactating village women. Status with regard to menstruation and ovulation was estimated on the basis of hormonal changes. The studies gave no information on infant supplementation, however. Maternal supplementation produced lower prolactin levels but no improvement in milk volume or frequency of breast-feeding (McNeilly *et al.*, 1981). Other studies report similar findings of lower PRL levels and milk yield. Even after 30 months, milk production was sustained with lower PRL until suckling frequency declined (Hennart *et al.*, 1981). Supplemented mothers had significantly shorter periods of postpartum amenorrhea and anovulation and higher pregnancy rates after 18 months (McNeilly *et al.*, 1981). The authors note that other studies had found no difference in postpartum fecundity between the poorly and well-nourished, but the supplements provided women in their study were significantly larger than those reported elsewhere. Questions on these findings remain since infant supplementation was not addressed nor was the possibility that the less well-nourished women might have had longer breast-feeding episodes or more frequent suckling (Prema *et al.*, 1979).

The Gambian studies estimated the impact of maternal nutritional status on postpartum fecundity and fertility to be a six-month decrease in the length of postpartum amenorrhea with improved nutritional status and an increase in conceptions from 19.2 percent of 180 conceptions occurring before 18 months postpartum to 33 percent of 54 conceptions. Studies in Guatemala (Delgado *et al.*, 1978) noted a difference in mean postpartum amenorrhea of 1.6 months between high and low nutritional status groups as defined by weight; and one month as defined by caloric intakes. Studies in Bangladesh reported differences in postpartum amenorrhea of 1.1 months (Chowdhury, 1978) using weight for height and 2.4 months (Huffman *et al.*, 1978) comparing the best- with the worst-nourished lactating women. McNeilly and colleagues (1981) estimate up to six months or more of infecundity in well-nourished, fully breast-feeding women. Undernourished mothers, who tend to breast-feed for a longer duration, may have two years of infecundity, even if the child begins supplementary foods from three to six months of age.

The significance of the effect of maternal malnutrition on postpartum infecundity has been carefully examined. Huffman *et al.* (1978, 1985) note that the nutritional effect on birth intervals and additional births would be on the order of less than one-tenth and less than one respectively. Bongaarts (1980), in his examination of data from Guatemala and Bangladesh, estimates a change in fertility rates of approximately 3 percent associated with improvement in maternal nutritional status. Convincing evidence of an inverse nutritional effect on the length of postpartum infecundity has been presented from Bangladesh and the Gambia (Huffman *et al.*, 1985; Lunn, 1982). Current debate centers around the significance and magnitude of its demographic impact. A joint committee of the WHO/NRL (1983) concluded that the relationship between maternal nutritional status and duration of lactational infecundity had "little demographic importance" since even substantial differences in maternal nutritional status could account for very little difference in infecundity. We feel that the research of Lunn *et al.* (e.g., 1981) in Gambia and the more recent research of Huffman *et al.* (1985) raise the possibility of a larger nutritional effect which may be demographically significant in high-fertility, poor countries such as Bangladesh.

Coital Frequency, Breast-feeding, and Fertility

Few studies have systematically examined the relationship of breast-feeding to coital frequency. The majority have looked at the phenomenon of postpartum abstinence, largely limited to traditional agrarian societies in tropical Africa and the Pacific. The reported reasons for the practice include folk beliefs (e.g., semen poisons breast milk) and more pragmatic concerns about maternal and child health. In most of these societies women abstain and men have other sexual outlets through polygynous marriages, extramarital relationships, or prostitution (Liskin, 1981).

Studies in Indonesia (Hull, 1978; Singarimbun and Manning, 1976) and in Nigeria (Caldwell and Caldwell, 1977) have documented postpartum abstinence prior to infant weaning. Similar practices have been reported in other areas of Africa and the Pacific. Traditional abstinence is disappearing as extended breast-feeding declines in urban and rural areas, particularly in East and Southern Africa, less so in West Africa (Liskin, 1981). Moreover, in regions where traditional taboos appear strongest, such as Indonesia, postpartum abstinence is now practiced much less frequently among the young (Hull, 1984).

Potentially important physiological effects of breast-feeding may be associated with reduced coital behavior. Adler and Cox (1983) examined the occurrence of depression among artificial- and breast-feeding mothers who may or may not have been also taking oral contraceptives. This prospective study of 89 postdelivery women found that among women not using oral contraceptives who breast-fed their infants, those who totally breast-fed had a significantly higher incidence of postnatal depression. Problems with the study included selection bias in which mothers more likely to be depressed may have chosen to breast-feed fully. The findings were difficult to interpret since there were relatively small numbers in each category, broken down into pill/nonpill, total/partial breast-feeding, and artificial feeders. No measure of coitus was available in the study report.

Coital frequency may be influenced by breast-feeding in several ways. The Adler and Cox (1983) study of depression indirectly supports the hypothesis that breast-feeding mothers might be more likely to have postnatal depression and may choose to curtail coitus postpartum. Anecdotal reports consistently describe breast-feeding mothers as often fatigued, which could also affect coital frequency. Traditional postpartum abstinence in some cultures is also reported. However, differences in the length of the abstinence as well as in compliance with the custom have been noted, even within study populations (Liskin, 1981), and postpartum abstinence will exert its effect on fertility variably among and within populations depending on how strictly and consistently it is practiced.

CONCLUSIONS

Breast-feeding is associated with a delay in the return of postpartum fecundity. Characteristics of breast-feeding performance importantly influence this relationship. Partial breast-feeding leads to longer periods of postpartum amenorrhea and anovulation than not breast-feeding, but to significantly shorter amenorrhea and ovulation than that associated with full breast-feeding. Breast-feeding duration, length and distribution in 24-hour feeding episodes, intensity of suckling and timing, rate of increase and type of supplement are additional characteristics that appear to be important. The mechanism by which lactation influences the return of postpartum fecundity appears to operate through the infant's suckling stimulus, which triggers a neurohormonal response that suppresses the return of fecundity postpartum. Confounding variables in relation to the outcome variable, fertility, include use of contraceptives and coital frequency. Other confounders may be maternal age and smoking status. Some studies show maternal nutritional status significantly influencing postpartum fecundity; others do not. More recent work indicates that the extent of supplementation of maternal diets may be critical in whether maternal nutritional status significantly affects postpartum fecundity. Research controlling all known confounding variables is needed to verify these findings. Evidence for a substantial negative effect of improved maternal nutritional status on postpartum fecundity is still lacking.

In spite of the consistency of findings about the fecundity-suppressing effect of lactation, several questions remain. Although longer breast-feeding is associated with longer infecundity, there is considerable variation in the duration of infecundity with a given duration of breast-feeding among populations and even among individuals within populations. This difference is only partially explained by suckling and less so by nutritional differences (McCann *et al.*, 1981). Improved research design including model specification, type of data collected, and analysis techniques based on known biological phenomena should provide more precision in the determination and quantification of effects (Habicht *et al.*, 1985).

9
INFANT FEEDING
AND THE HOUSEHOLD

THEORETICAL PATHWAYS

The process of feeding an infant affects not only the intimately involved infant and mother, but may also significantly affect the entire household. The household can be thought of as a complex ecological system, in which change in one component throws the system out of balance, necessitating readjustments in other components until a new balance is achieved. As figure IX-1 illustrates, infant feeding can directly affect two components of the household system: expenditures and time. Because of the complex relationships among components of the system, changes in these two components can bring about changes in many others. Some of these secondary changes may be immediate and obvious, others may be long term and subtle. Some of the changes may be detrimental to the welfare of household members, others beneficial, and still others neutral. Some changes are more readily quantifiable than others. The following aspects are more amenable to study.

The first major pathway in this system involves the effect of infant feeding on household expenditures. The net effect can be broken down into cost of the goods involved in feeding (food and equipment) and changes that may occur in purchase of other goods and services which compensate, to some extent, for the cost of goods. The net result is that additional cash outlay for infant feeding may be considerably less than the cost of feeding-related goods, but the purchase of other goods and services may be affected. Part of the cost of goods may be met by decreasing the amount of food available to other household members, by buying a less expensive mix of food, or by changing expenditures on other budget items.

The second pathway operates through the effect of infant feeding on allocation of time of household members to various activities. Since time is always a limited commodity, that required for infant feeding necessitates reallocation of time use by the mother and other household members. Infant

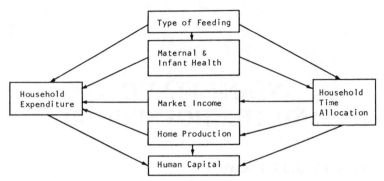

FIGURE IX-1   Effects of infant feeding on household expenditures and time.

feeding can affect the time allocation of other household members directly if they assume some responsibility for feeding. Household time is affected indirectly if, because of increased demands on the mother's time, tasks she previously performed are taken over by other household members. Similar changes in the time allocation of other household members can occur if someone other than the mother assumes infant-feeding responsibilities.

Changes in household time allocation can affect money income by altering the amount of time spent in market production. Changes in the allocation of time can also affect the time spent in home production of child care, food, etc. Alterations in cash income and home production will in turn affect expenditures.

The type of feeding may also influence the infant's health (see part 2) which, in turn, can affect household expenditures and time allocation. If one type of feeding produces a less healthy infant, more time and money may be spent caring for the infant than would be spent for an infant fed by another method. Type of feeding may also affect the mother's health (see part 3), which may have an impact on her time allocation and earnings.

Finally, allocation of time and expenditures may affect the development of human capital of household members. For example, children might be taken out of school to feed infant siblings or to perform other home or market production activities previously carried out by the mother. Increased demands on a mother's time can decrease the time she devotes to child care which, if not compensated for by someone else's time, can have a negative effect on the children's development. The increased cost of food for infant feeding may be met by decreasing expenditures on food or health care for other family members, to their detriment.

A few studies have investigated the cost of goods used in infant feeding. Fewer have analyzed the amount of time different feeding methods require. No studies have looked at the reallocations that may occur in other household uses of time and money. Although time and money costs may be significantly different for different feeding methods, it is not clear how the household reacts to these costs or whether the net effects after reallocations are significantly different.

The impact of infant feeding on the household varies with age of the infant. First, the type of food changes with age, from breast milk to other milks to solids. Second, as the infant develops, the mode of feeding changes, with the infant ultimately feeding itself. These changes can have a dramatic effect on the time and money the household requires.

We are considering two separate hypotheses in this book. Discussion of either hypothesis involves reference to the same general pathways outlined above. Under both hypotheses, different feeding methods are expected to have different levels of impact on the household. The alternative hypotheses, however, incorporate somewhat different issues and methodological problems and are discussed separately.

METHODOLOGICAL ISSUES

In this section we discuss some of the methodological issues involved in investigating the effect of infant feeding on the household and the pathways represented in figure IX-1.

Data

A major methodological issue in investigating effects of infant feeding on the household concerns the use of actual data or hypothetical calculations, based on nutrient requirements and average costs of different foods. Most previous research has relied heavily on the latter, incorporating many unfounded assumptions (see the review at the end of this section), with the result that conclusions do not necessarily reflect real household behavior.

Policy decisions should ideally be based on actual behavior, but relevant behavioral information is often difficult and costly to collect.

Care must be taken in interpreting the results of a comparative analysis of true money and time costs of different feeding methods. Hypothetical calculations generally assume that, for whatever feeding methods are used, mothers and infants receive an adequate quality and quantity of food, thus reducing the possibility of significant health differences according to feeding method. In developing countries mothers and infants may not receive adequate nutrition, and possibly the level of inadequacy is related to the type of feeding (see chapters 5 and 7). Thus, significant health differences are likely between breast-feeding mother-infant pairs and those with children fed other foods. The true costs of each method must include quantification of these health differences.

Extensive literature on the methodology of measuring and valuing health will not be reviewed here. Although in practice it is difficult to place a value on differences in health, the possibility of such differences should be kept in mind when comparing actual expenditures and time costs of different feeding methods.

Expenditures

The effect of infant feeding on household expenditures includes the cost of the goods involved in infant feeding and the compensatory changes in the household's expenditures pattern. Ultimately, data on these two components will indicate the household resources allocated to infant feeding and the net impact on the household's expenditure patterns.

Goods costs

In the case of breast-feeding, the amount the household spends on food and equipment used for infant feeding is the cost of additional food for the mother. Because all household food is generally purchased at the same time, and an increase in food for the mother may be counteracted by decreased food for other members, changes in household food expenditures will not necessarily reflect the cost of additional food. A more appropriate measure would be to observe changes in the mother's intake because of lactation and cost out the differences.

The money cost of feeding with other foods includes the cost of food, special equipment, and additional fuel used for preparing the food. It is relatively easy to measure the cost of special infant foods not consumed by other household members. If the infant is eating some adult foods, consumption of those foods must be measured and costed as was suggested for lactating mothers. The major equipment for artificial feeding is usually bottles and nipples, although cup and spoon feeding may be practiced in some areas. The purchase of other items, such as an extra cooking pot, should be considered in cost analyses, but such items are not expected to add substantially to the cost of feeding. Because the cost of all equipment is spread over the life of each item, resulting daily costs may be negligible. Use of additional fuel is difficult to measure and value, and the resulting costs may not be practically significant. Studies of small samples may indicate whether fuel costs should be examined in larger investigations.

Specification of the independent variable, type of feeding, will depend on dependent variables being considered. In the case of the cost of goods, the type of feeding can be measured as a continuous variable, expressed as the contribution of breast milk or other foods to the total infant diet. Because the nutrient density of other foods varies, simply measuring the volume of other foods may not give an accurate picture of their contribution to the diet. The actual nutrient content of each feeding method is a more appropriate measure of their contribution. The choice of which nutrients to measure will depend on the situation.

Other environmental factors influence the cost of infant feeding and must be controlled for. The existence of certain assets, usually strongly related to socioeconomic status, such as a refrigerator that allows purchase of food in bulk quantities at lower cost and proper storage of leftovers, will affect costs.

The availability of time of household members may influence the degree to which more expensive commercially prepared foods are used instead of time-intensive home prepared foods.

Pattern of expenditures

There is no *a priori* reason to believe that type of infant feeding has an independent effect on selection of compensatory budget items. However, the relative magnitudes of changes in budget items are likely to vary depending on feeding methods. It would be desirable not only to describe changes in the pattern of expenditures, but to rank them according to their impact on the household. Such a ranking system is difficult to develop. While a decrease in food purchasing is generally considered more harmful to human well-being than a decrease in entertainment expenditures, it is less clear whether it is more harmful than a decrease in health care expenditures. Without such a ranking system, investigations on this subject must be restricted to describing changes in the mix of goods and services the household purchases.

Choice of the appropriate measure of the change in goods and services depends on the category being investigated. The amount of money spent on a certain category is a convenient means of quantification, but it ignores the possibility that the household may be able to increase its efficiency and procure the same quantity and quality of a good or service at a lower price.

Two useful dimensions for classifying household purchases are by major budget items, such as food and shelter, and household member. Ideally, both dimensions should be investigated. Determining goods and services purchased for each person is more difficult than examining all items purchased, because expenditures may be for items shared by several household members. However, the amount of food available to each member is likely to be strongly affected by infant feeding, and should therefore be studied carefully.

Changes in the household pattern of expenditures are related to costs incurred through infant feeding, which are in turn related to the contribution of each feeding method to the infant's total diet. Therefore, the independent variable, infant-feeding method, should be specified in terms of the percentage of nutrient intake each method contributes.

A variety of factors is likely to play a strong role in the household's decisions on how to alter its budget to compensate for infant feeding. Cultural norms will likely influence which household members and budget categories are most affected. Socioeconomic status may similarly be significant. Wealthier households may be able to allocate more funds to infant feeding from luxury items than can poorer households.

Time

Three issues need to be considered with regard to the effects of infant feeding on time: (1) the absolute amount of time involved in each method, (2) the reallocation of time among household members, and (3) the cost or value of these changes in time.

Amount of time

The time necessary for breast-feeding and for feeding with other foods can differ considerably. Of interest is the amount of time spent in all aspects of each feeding method. Theoretically, the total time for breast-feeding includes that spent procuring, preparing, and eating the extra food required by the mother, as well as the time the mother and infant spend eating. Total time inputs to other feeding methods include feeding time plus time spent procuring and preparing food and equipment.

Since, for mixed-feeding, time inputs can be allocated to each feeding method, the independent variable, type of feeding, can be measured as a continuous variable. The amount of time spent on each feeding method as a percentage of total time used for infant feeding is the appropriate measure of the independent variable.

The effect of each feeding method on total time inputs is affected by possession of certain assets. The type of cooking equipment used can affect the amount of time necessary for preparing food for mother and infant. Similarly, a readily available supply of potable water eliminates the need to boil water for use in preparing concentrated infant foods.

Reallocation of time

Since time is a limited commodity in any household, the time demands of infant feeding will notably cause reallocations in time use by many household members.

No attempt will be made here to rank allocation schemes. Of greater interest is a description of changes in time devoted to major tasks, such as market production, child care, and other home production activities.

Significant differences in characteristics of the activities involved in each feeding method modify their effects on the time inputs of various household members. Although breast-feeding requires a heavy investment of a mother's time, it does not require her undivided attention; she can perform other tasks simultaneously. Economists term this *joint production*. In many societies, a substantial amount of breast-feeding takes place at night, and does not greatly interfere with a mother's sleep. Thus, the amount of other household members' time required to fill the gap left by the demands of breast-feeding on the mother's time may be less than the total number of hours an infant spends suckling.

Artificial feeding allows for a wider range of involvement of other household members in the feeding process. At one extreme, the mother still performs all feeding-related tasks, or other household members can assume some or all feeding responsibilities, freeing the mother's time for other activities. At the other extreme, at a certain stage of development, the infant can feed itself by being propped up with a bottle, although an older person must prepare the food and supervise the feeding. In contrast to breast-feeding, the preparation and feeding tasks associated with other feeding methods generally do not allow other tasks to be performed at the same time.

As in the previous case, the independent variable, infant-feeding method, can be specified in terms of the amount of time spent in each feeding method as a percentage of total infant-feeding time.

Other factors than type of feeding also affect reallocation of household members' time. For example, the relative educational level of household members affects their wage-earning potential and, thus, the allocation of their time among various activities. These and other confounding factors must be taken into consideration in any comparison of time inputs of different feeding methods.

Value of time

In comparing the effects of infant-feeding methods on household time allocation, attempts are often made to place a value on time. Measuring the value of time is a complex issue which will not be discussed in depth. However, a few issues specific to the valuation of infant-feeding time need to be considered. One is the recognition that other household members may be involved in other feeding methods and that the value of their time may be different from that of the mother. A second concerns the relative value of a person's time at different times of the day. Time is often valued according to an individual's actual or potential market wage rate. Feeding takes place throughout a 24-hour period, and the value of time at night, when wage labor may be unavailable, is probably different from its value during the day. A third issue concerns joint production—performing other tasks simultaneously with feeding, which may be especially significant in relation to breast-feeding. Joint production would reduce the value of time spent feeding. If joint production does occur, consideration must be given to the relative efficiency of a mother's performance of other tasks while feeding.

Income

One way of valuing the time costs of infant feeding is to determine the effects of different feeding methods on income. Because each feeding method has different time requirements and characteristics, different feeding methods will probably have varied effects on income. Of interest in this regard is the change in household income associated with the pattern of infant feeding. Several factors must be considered when measuring income changes. Because the time of other household members may be substituted for the mother's time in the market place, an increase in their earnings may compensate for a decrease in her earnings. Considering a change in the mother's income only would overstate the effect on total household income. Breast-feeding is not necessarily incompatible with market production. The effect on mother's income cannot be evaluated simply by multiplying the hours devoted to infant feeding by her wage rate. If calculations of the effect of feeding on income are made in the absence of data collection, some consideration must be given to the availability of work. Because of high unemployment rates, every woman who is home feeding an infant may not be able to find a market job even if she wants one.

Since the effects of infant feeding on income are related to the amount of time spent feeding, the independent variable describing feeding should be measured in units of time.

The effects of feeding on income are likely to be confounded by several factors. The nature of the labor market of which each household is a part is perhaps the most significant factor. Socioeconomic status, household size, other working household members, and educational levels of members may also affect changes in income independently and must be controlled for.

Home Production

Economists use the term *home production* to refer to use of the time of household members to produce goods and services which could alternatively be purchased in the market place. The basic concept is that time can be used to earn income which then purchases goods and services, or, alternatively, time is used to produce the goods and services directly. Such home-produced goods and services include producing, processing, and preparing food, and providing child care. Because infant feeding usually involves the mother more than other household members, and she is often the one most involved in home production, different feeding methods are likely to have a significant impact on the level and mix of home production.

The outcome variable in the analysis of home production should be measured in terms of changes in the value of home-produced goods and services. However, since valuing such activities is difficult, changes can be measured in the amount of time spent in various home production activities. Since the effects of infant feeding on home production are related to the broader question of time allocation, the independent variable for this analysis should be categorized on the basis of the amount of time spent in different feeding methods.

A number of factors related to socioeconomic status may confound the relationship between infant feeding and home production. Having certain assets may make production activities sufficiently efficient that the same quantity and quality of goods and services can be produced with smaller inputs of time. Likewise, skill levels of household members may affect their efficiency in home production.

Human Capital

Development of human capital refers to improvement in a person's ability to function productively in society. Education and health care are specific activities which add to human capital. Although the entity itself is difficult to measure (e.g., knowledge or health status), inputs to the creation of human capital can be measured. Examples include the adequacy of dietary intake, the amount of time spent with children in developmental activities, level of schooling, and use of preventive and curative health care measures, all of which can be affected by infant feeding.

Infant and Maternal Health

The effect of differences in maternal and infant health on expenditures can be measured in terms of the actual cost of health care and the reallocations that may occur in other household expenditures. The significant components of the impact of need for health care on household time include the amount of time spent providing care to an unhealthy infant or mother, plus changes which may occur in allocation of the mother's time because of changes in her health. If either of these changes results in a change in market production, income is likely to be affected as well.

REVIEW OF STUDIES

Limited research has been conducted on the impact of infant feeding on the household. Some information is available concerning goods and time costs, but no studies have investigated how households react to these costs. Table IX-1 summarizes information on time and goods costs of infant feeding in studies conducted in developing countries.

With the exception of the research by Popkin (1978) and the information on feeding time incorporated into the study by Greiner et al. (1979), all studies calculated relative costs on the basis of hypothetical information. None goes beyond determining time and goods costs to examine how costs of infant feeding affect household resource allocation.

The study by Greiner et al. (1979) incorporates the most extensive definition of costs, including estimates for components other than food in calculating goods costs and feeding time in calculating time costs. Although calculating time inputs resulted in the somewhat surprising conclusion that other feeding methods are three to four times more time intensive than breast-feeding, a number of problems with the method of calculation make these results questionable. The sample of mothers for whom breast-feeding times are measured includes women who are only partially breast-feeding. The time figures reported thus underestimate the true time required for exclusive breast-feeding. Although data were collected on several components of time required for other feeding methods, Greiner et al. felt that the actual time spent in preparation was inadequate to ensure a safe product. To compensate for this supposed deficit, the study used hypothetical figures two to three times greater than actual observations. Finally, the total time required for other feeding methods included an estimate of time required for caring for a sick infant which was significantly greater than the estimate for caring for a breast-fed infant. Since the study assumed that an adequate quantity and quality of other foods were being fed, inclusion of a substantial time cost for added health care for artifically fed infants is questionable.

The Popkin study (1978) collected data and thus provides a more realistic

TABLE IX-1

Effect of infant feeding on expenditure and time

Study	Study Notes	Cost of Goods ($/day)				Time Costs (minutes & $/day)							Conclusions/ Comments
		Breast-feeding	Other feeding methods			Breast-feeding			Other feeding methods				
		Mother's food	Food	Other	Total	Feeding	Other	Total	Feeding	Prep	Other	Total	
McKigney, 1971 Jamaica	Hypothetical (extra 1000 kcal/day)	.08 – .54	.11 – .42	—	—								OFM: greater goods costs, no time costs
Villa-Real, 1975, Philippines	Hypothetical (extra 1000 kcal/day)	.123 – .473[a]	46 – 01[a]	—	.246 – .301[a]	90.0							OFM: greater goods costs, no time costs. Considered work/BF compatibility in valuing time
Popkin, 1978 Philippines	N = 33 BF; 17 OF poor rich[b]	.024[a] .127[a]	124[a] 67[a]	.002[a] .003[a]	.126[a] .170[a]	68.6 16.3	— —	68.6 $0.073[a] 116.3 $0.146[a]	22.0 29.1	— —	— —	22.0 $0.057[a] 29.1 $0.147[a]	OFM: total time costs more for poor, similar for rich; BF time intensive—OFM goods intensive. OFM time costs exclude preparation time

TABLE IX-1 (continued)

Study	Study Notes	Cost of Goods ($/day)				Time Costs (minutes & $/day)							Conclusions/ Comments
		Breast-feeding	Other feeding methods			Breast-feeding			Other feeding methods				
		Mother's food	Food	Other	Total	Feed-ing	Other	Total	Feed-ing	Prep	Other	Total	
Greiner et al., 1979, Ghana & Ivory Coast	Actual feeding time—remainder hypothetical	.07– .14	.26– .37	.183 (equip-ment & fuel)	.42– .53	48 40.1	7.1 8.5	55.1 $0.34 48.6	27 27	90 135	15.4 39.1	132.4 $0.64 201.1 $0.90	Avg family saves $491–723 (excluding disease cost) in 2 yrs BF. Unjustifiable assumptions on BF time involvement; see text

Notes: BF = breast-fed/breast-feeding; OF = fed other foods; OFM = other feeding methods

[a]based on conversion: 7.35 pesos = $1.00

[b]Adding 1000 extra kcal/day = poor, .118[a]; no change for rich

picture. The results are based on two days of observation in each of three different seasons. However, time inputs for other feeding methods included only actual feeding time. Without information on preparation time for other feeding methods, comparisons of the time inputs for the two methods can lead to erroneous conclusions.

A major problem in those studies which investigate time costs of infant feeding is related to the measurement and valuation of time. Studies which collect data on time generally ignore the joint production discussed earlier. Most studies consider all time spent feeding to be time not spent in other activities. One data set on joint production comes from a small observational study of rural households in the Philippines. Jayme-Ho (1976) found that the two mothers in the sample who were breast-feeding spent a total of 17.8 hours per week in breast-feeding as a primary activity and an additional hour per week in secondary activity. When breast-feeding was the primary activity, these mothers were often engaged in other, secondary activities, though the actual figures and activities for the latter are not reported. In time allocation studies carried out in Africa, child care and rearing are often not counted since African families rarely perform them alone (Berio, 1984).

A second problem in estimating time costs relates to the practice of applying an average wage rate to all time spent feeding, ignoring the different values time has at different times of day. The study by Villa-Real (1975) addressed this issue by assuming that only four of the average nine feedings per day took place during working hours, and applied the average wage rate only to time spent on those four feedings.

Two studies have investigated the distribution of time spent in other feeding methods by all household members plus hired help. Table IX-2 summarizes the results. Although the breakdown varies by culture and socioeconomic status, it is clear that a significant proportion of the feeding of other foods is performed by persons other than the mother.

The only information on the impact of infant feeding on household food intakes comes from data Arroyave (1976) provided from Latin America. In all six countries surveyed, for the family as a unit, dietary intakes were more often inadequate in families with lactating women than in those with neither pregnant nor lactating women (see table IX-3). While this information is suggestive that lactation has a detrimental effect on dietary intakes of other household members, it is certainly not conclusive. The higher percentage of inadequate family intakes may have been because of differences in the mothers' diets, with intakes of other members remaining

TABLE IX-2

Percentage of time various household members spend in infant feeding

Study	Mother	Father	Other children	Other relatives	Maid
Greiner *et al.*, 1979 Ghana, N = 13; urban					
% of feedings	39.0	12.0		16.0[a]	33.0
Popkin, 1978 Philippines, N = 17; rural					
% of feeding time:					
poor	53.3	28.2	19.5	0	0
rich	47.8	7.9	8.9	35.4	0

[a]Grandmother

TABLE IX-3

Adequacy[a] of calorie intake of rural families with lactating women compared to those without—1965–67

Country	Families with lactating women	Families without pregnant or lactating women
Costa Rica	37	28
El Salvador	26	16
Guatemala	18	12
Honduras	43	31
Nicaragua	49	24
Panama	36	15

Source: Arroyave, 1976.
[a]Percentage of families with adequacy less than 75 percent of weighted recommended allowances

unchanged. Information on adequacy of the family diet that excludes the mother's is needed to draw any conclusions.

The only conclusion that can be reached from these studies is that the goods costs of breast-feeding appears, at least theoretically, to be less than those of other feeding methods, especially for the poor. The situation regarding time is not so clear. In these studies, the amount of time spent breast-feeding ranged from 48.6 to 90 minutes per day while the range for other feeding methods was from 22 to 201 minutes per day. Such a wide variation in results, combined with the methodological problems discussed above, precludes drawing conclusions and indicates a strong need for further research.

EFFECTS ON THE HOUSEHOLD OF FEEDING INFANTS OTHER FOODS

A wide variety of foods and feeding methods are used throughout the world to feed infants, ranging from gruels to powdered skim milk-based mixtures to prepared commercial formulas. Methods range from bottle-feeding to cup-feeding to self-feeding. Each combination of food and method will probably require different inputs of time and money and have a different impact on the household. Only by studying combinations of method and food can the effects of various patterns be determined.

Methodological Issues

Expenditures

In calculating the goods cost of other feeding routines, care must be taken to include all cost components. The cost of the food itself will usually vary widely because of different levels of embedded time and fuel costs. Highly prepared foods may cost more money but require less preparation time. Preparing infant food at home may require the purchase of special equipment whereas buying commercially prepared foods can eliminate this cost. Bottle-feeding requires the purchase of bottles and nipples, but cup-feeding can be done with utensils generally in the household.

Time

Feeding methods other than breast-feeding may differ significantly in both preparation and feeding times. Home-prepared infant foods require considerably more time to prepare than commercial foods. Cup-feeding may require different inputs of time than bottle-feeding. Different feeding routines may require different levels of skill and training. The level of skill required may influence which household members feed the infant, and thus affect the total allocation of their time. The time and skill inputs necessary for feeding will vary not only with the feeding method, but also with the age of the infant.

Review of Studies

Many studies conducted on the cost of breast-feeding versus other feeding methods have examined the hypothetical goods costs of different types of feeding methods. McKigney (1968) calculated a range of cost in the West Indies from $0.125 for 1,000 kcal provided by skim milk powder to $0.40 for milk-based infant formula to $2.44 for commercial strained meats. In Jamaica, McKigney (1972) found a range of from $0.11 per day for a home-prepared infant formula consisting of reconstituted skim milk powder, vegetable oil, sugar, and vitamins to $0.37 per day for commercial infant formula. In the Ivory Coast, Greiner et al. (1979) calculated that a feeding routine based on commercial infant formula for the first four months followed by full cream powdered milk for the remainder of the first year resulted in an average daily cost of $0.26, while feeding commercial infant formula for an entire year would cost $0.371 per day.

Popkin and Latham (1973) calculated the cost of several commercial, low-cost, nutritious foods and indigenous multimixes promoted as supplementary foods for infants. Calculations based on their cost information reveal a range of $0.327 to $0.891 per day to meet the caloric requirements of an infant with commercially prepared foods, and $0.010 to $0.017 per day for home-prepared multimixes.

All of these results are based on the cost of food alone and do not consider differences in equipment or fuel costs. We found no study which estimated, much less collected data on, the time costs of different artificial feeding methods.

Based on this limited information, there appears to be a wide range in estimated costs of food used in other feeding methods. No conclusions can be drawn about other goods costs or time costs. Considering the wide range of other infant foods available in developing countries, much more research needs to be conducted on foods actually used, in what quantities, and at what cost in time and money.

CONCLUSIONS

Very little attention has been focused on the effects of various infant-feeding methods on household members other than the infant and the mother. Theoretically, different feeding routines can have substantially different impacts on the allocation of both household time and money. Before recommendations are made endorsing one feeding regimen over another, effects on the household must be considered along with effects on the infant and the mother.

10
THE INFANT-FEEDING TRIAD

In this book we have laid out theoretical pathways by which infant feeding could affect a variety of outcomes, reviewed previous biological and epidemiological research concerning these pathways in an effort to assess the current level of knowledge, identified research gaps, and developed research hypotheses. Special attention has been given to identifying underlying methodological problems which have limited the value of previous research. Our approach to this subject is unique in two ways: we consider the effects of infant feeding on the mother and the household as well as on the infant and the effects of a wide range of foods fed to infants, rather than limiting the discussion only to breast milk or commercial infant formula.

A major methodological issue in research on infant feeding is appropriate specification of different feeding methods. A particular feeding pattern can be described by a number of attributes—frequency of feeding, duration of a single feeding, quantity of nutrients ingested, for example. Which attributes are used to describe different methods depends on the outcomes investigated and practical considerations of data collection. We have discussed different outcomes of infant feeding and have been careful to identify the most appropriate means of specifying infant-feeding methods in analyzing each outcome.

In discussing the impact of infant feeding on the infant, we have focused on two separate but related pathways, one involving the effects on morbidity and mortality through effects of feeding on the immunologic system. The second pathway concerned effects on infant growth through the effect of feeding on nutritional status.

There is considerable evidence that breast milk may affect the infant's immunologic system in ways other foods cannot. An infant's immunologic system is less mature than that of an adult. Between four to six months of age, immunologic elements received during gestation have fallen to a low level, and the infant may not yet be able to produce its own protection to replace this loss. Thus, the four-to-six-month-old infant may be more susceptible to infection than younger or older infants. Breast milk contains a variety of immunologic elements which may provide much needed protection, especially during this period. Breast-fed infants may also be exposed to fewer pathogens than infants fed other foods. However, it is not clear how the immunologic factors in breast milk function, since they are unlikely to be absorbed intact. It is thought that the immunologic elements in breast milk provide local protection in the gut, either eliminating pathogens before they can be absorbed into the system or changing the gut environment to make it unfavorable for the growth of pathogens. This local effect suggests that persistence of the immunologic benefit of breast milk should not be expected once breast-feeding has ceased and the immunologic elements have been degraded. It also suggests that breast-feeding most benefits the infant by protecting it against pathogens which affect the gut and the upper respiratory tract.

Epidemiologic evidence tends to agree with the immunologic evidence that nonbreast-fed infants generally experience significantly more morbidity and mortality than breast-fed infants. This finding has been consistent despite research use of differing methodologies, definitions of morbidity, causes of mortality, and study populations. A variety of methodological issues prevent more precise quantification of the effect of breast-feeding on morbidity and mortality, and limit our ability to characterize the relationship further between breast-feeding and morbidity and mortality. While epidemiological indices indicate that the peak benefits of breast-feeding seem to occur between three and nine months of age, it is not yet possible to assess the relationship between supplementation and morbidity and mortality, and possible long-term effects of breast-feeding after the practice ceases. The studies are also inadequate for evaluating hypotheses regarding other foods and morbidity.

Besides its effect on morbidity, infant feeding also affects an infant's growth. Several serious methodological problems arise in investigating the effects of feeding on infant growth. Contrary to what is found with morbidity, nutrient intakes and growth can be excessive as well as deficient. There is a theoretical optimal level of nutrient intake or growth, somewhere between the two extremes. Standards developed attempt to identify optimal nutrient intakes and optimal growth, but there is controversy over their validity and application in low-income countries. Nutrient intake and growth standards have generally been based on observations of intakes of healthy breast-fed or bottle-fed infants, rather than on any set of functional or developmental criteria.

A second major methodological problem involves quantifying intakes. The ability of any food to sustain growth is related to the quantity ingested and its nutrient composition. Most previous studies on infant feeding and growth have not adequately controlled for quantity or quality of infant food, especially of breast milk. New techniques for measuring breast milk quantity are needed especially for use under field conditions, and on other more easily measured variables which correlate highly with breast milk production and can be used as proxies (e.g., maternal body fat composition).

Some research, based on theoretical calculations of infant nutrient requirements and observations on apparent limitations to breast milk production, has indicated that exclusive breast-feeding may provide insufficient energy to support adequate growth beyond three or four months of age. Whether the amounts and quality of other foods fed to infants in low-income countries can theoretically promote growth for as long or longer has not been investigated. Human milk differs considerably from commercial formula and other milks in the amounts and forms of its biochemical components. However, these compositional differences are not expected to have a pronounced effect on growth (although they may affect other developmental processes) so long as adequate quantities of essential nutrients are provided.

Epidemiological studies comparing growth of infants fed different foods have been inconclusive, in part because of methodological problems discussed above. In high-income countries, exclusive breast-feeding appears to support adequate growth for at least the first six months, but whether it supports "better" growth than feeding other foods is not known. The situation in low-income countries is not clear. Few studies have controlled for confounding variables such as morbidity and birth weight; or have measured the quantities of foods ingested by infants. Most studies have been cross-sectional rather than longitudinal.

Although we treat morbidity and nutritional status (as reflected by growth) as separate outcomes of infant feeding, they are, in fact, related. Morbidity has been shown to affect nutritional status through changes in feeding patterns and metabolic changes, and nutritional status can affect morbidity through a variety of mechanisms leading to decreased resistance to infection. When studying the effect of infant feeding on either outcome, the other consequence must be controlled for as a confounding variable, and consideration given to the interactions between the two relationships.

Infant feeding can affect the mother in two ways: it can affect her nutritional status and her fertility. Nutritional status can be affected by changes in nutrient supplies through changes in dietary intake and stores and through changes in metabolic demands of breast-feeding and physical activity. Maternal nutritional status is most obviously affected by breast-feeding because of the increased nutrient demands of milk production. How lactating women in low-income countries meet these nutrient demands is not known. Their breast milk production may be lower than that of well-nourished high-income women, but the process requires a substantial amount of additional energy and other nutrients. The dietary intake of women in low-income countries rarely meets recommended levels for lactation (especially for energy), and is usually not significantly higher than that of nonpregnant, nonlactating counterparts. Although lactating women do lose weight, indicating the use of stored energy, it is not clear whether their weight loss exceeds stores laid down during pregnancy, or whether this weight loss is permanent and cumulative with repeated periods of lactation. It is also not known whether the level of physical activity of lactating women is different from that of nonlactating women.

Separate aspects of the effects of lactation on a mother's nutritional status have been investigated, but no one study has looked at the total situation to determine how women in low-income countries support the nutrient demands of lactation. Nor is information available on how other feeding methods affect maternal nutritional status. It is conceivable that the high cost of other foods may result in less food being available to the mother or an offsetting increase in her physical (wage-earning) activity, either of which may affect her nutritional status.

Infant feeding can affect fertility by three separate pathways. Breast-feeding may affect the frequency and intensity of infant suckling, which may affect levels of hormones that influence fecundity. Feeding may also affect maternal nutritional status which may have a direct impact on fecundity. Infant-feeding practices may also affect (interfere with) coital frequency.[1] Major difficulties arise in investigations of fecundity and fertility because of problems inherent in measuring variables. The exact return of fecundity is very difficult and costly to measure in field situations, so proxy measures are generally used, such as the return of menstruation and birth intervals. Aspects of infant feeding thought to be related to hormonal levels, such as suckling frequency and intensity are also not easily measured.

Previous research has shown that lactation is associated with longer delays in the return of menstruation and ovulation, and longer birth intervals than are the case with other feeding methods. Full breast-feeding has a

---

[1] A fourth pathway, the effect of breast-feeding on contraceptive use, is not addressed in this review although it certainly merits additional research.

stronger impact on these indicators of fecundity than partial breast-feeding. The results suggest that the most significant pathway is the effect of suckling frequency and intensity on hormonal levels. It is not clear whether maternal nutritional status also is involved in delaying the return of fecundity post-partum, and whether maternal nutritional status is affected differently by different infant-feeding methods. Cultural practices (taboos) are felt to limit postpartum coital frequency. There are also potential physiological effects of lactation which may affect coital frequency. These separate effects of lactation on coital frequency, and, in turn, of coital frequency on fertility have not been carefully investigated. To what extent do these taboos actually limit coital frequency? Are these practices limited to lactating women or applied to all postpartum women? To what extent are they actually followed within and across cultures?

The effects of infant feeding extend also to other members of the house-hold. Feeding requires expenditures of time and money, both of which have alternative uses within the household. Thus buying food, either for the lactating mother or the baby, or spending time in food purchasing and preparation as well as in actual feeding necessitates a reallocation of money and time from other household activities. How the household manages this reallocation is a major aspect of the overall effect of infant feeding on the household. The cost of additional food may be met by decreasing expenditures on other budget items such as food for other household members or health care, or it may cause an increase in market production by some household members. The time inputs to infant feeding may reduce the time available for other home production activities. Thus, cash income, home production, and development of the human capital of household members may all be affected by infant feeding.

Previous research in this area is scanty and fraught with methodological problems. Studies are often based on hypothetical calculations of what it would take to feed an infant or a lactating woman adequately rather than on direct observations of what households spend, in terms of time and money, on infant feeding. Such studies have rarely included all of the associated costs such as that of special equipment for preparing and feeding other infant foods and the time costs involved in purchasing and preparing foods for the mother or infant. Based on the available information, it appears that the cost of goods involved in feeding an infant other foods is higher than that of providing extra food to a lactating woman, and the costs of different other foods may vary widely. Which feeding method is the more time intensive is not clear, nor is there any information on time costs of other feeding methods. There is no information on how expenditures of money and time on infant feeding affect other aspects of the household, such as time available for market and home production or cash available for food, health care, or child education.

In summary, we have addressed a crucial subject, the consequences of infant feeding. Over the past decade this topic has been the focus of heated debate. Most of the debate, we feel, has centered narrowly on the consequences of breast-feeding on the infant, lumping together all other foods under the category of formula- or bottle-feeding. As a result, crucial distinctions in the types of other food infants consume have been ignored. Moreover the effects of infant feeding on the mother and the household have been largely unexplored. A refocus of research in this area on the effects of overall infant-feeding patterns, in particular of other infant foods on the triad—the infant, the mother, and the household—is needed.

BIBLIOGRAPHY

AAP. See American Academy of Pediatrics.

Abedin, Mehnur, and Charles H. Kirkpatrick (1980). Immunosuppressive activity of cord blood leukocytes. *Pediatrics* **66**, 405–410.

Acheson, K. J., I. T. Campbell, O. G. Edholm, D. S. Miller, and M. J. Stock (1980). The measurement of food and energy intake in man—An evaluation of some techniques. *American Journal of Clinical Nutrition* **33**, 1147–1154.

Adams, J. M., A. C. Kimball, and F. H. Adams (1947). Early immunization against pertussis. *American Journal of Diseases of Children* **74**, 10–18.

Adebonojo, Festus O. (1972). Artificial vs breast feeding. Relation to infant health in a middle class American community. *Clinical Pediatrics* **11**, 25–29.

Adler, Elizabeth M., and John L. Cox (1983). Breast feeding and post-natal depression. *Journal of Psychosomatic Research* **27**, 139–144.

Ahn, Chung Hae, and William C. MacLean, Jr. (1980). Growth of the exclusively breast-fed infant. *American Journal of Clinical Nutrition* **33**, 183–192.

Ainsworth, Mary D. Salter (1977). Infant development and mother-infant interaction among Ganda and American families. In *Culture and Infancy: Variations in the Human Experience*, edited by P. Herbert Leiderman, Steven R. Tulkin, and Anne Rosenfeld. The Child Psychology Series. Academic Press, New York, pp. 119–149.

Aitchison, J. M., W. L. Dunkley, N. L. Canolty, and L. M. Smith (1977). Influence of diet on trans fatty acids in human milk. *American Journal of Clinical Nutrition* **30**, 2006–2015.

Akin, John S., Charles C. Griffin, David K. Guilkey, and Barry M. Popkin (1985). Determinants of infant feeding: A household production approach. *Economic Development and Cultural Change* **34**, 57–81.

Akin, John S., Richard E. Bilsborrow, David K. Guilkey, Barry M. Popkin, Daniel Benoit, Pierre Cantrelle, Michele Garenne, and Pierre Levi (1981). The determinants of breast-feeding in Sri Lanka. *Demography* **18**, 287–307.

Allen, Lindsay H. (1982). Calcium bioavailability and absorption: A review. *American Journal of Clinical Nutrition* **35**, 783–808.

American Academy of Pediatrics (1979). Normal nutrition in infancy and childhood. *Pediatric Nutrition Handbook*. Evanston, Ill., pp. 91–157.

American Academy of Pediatrics, Committee on Nutrition (1976). Commentary on breast-feeding and infant formulas, including proposed standards for formulas. *Nutrition Reviews* **34**, 248–256.

American Academy of Pediatrics, Committee on Nutrition (1977). Nutritional needs of low-birth-weight infants. *Pediatrics* **60**, 519–530.

American Academy of Pediatrics, Committee on Nutrition (1985). Nutritional needs of low-birth-weight infants. *Pediatrics* **75**, 976–986.

Ammann, Arthur J., and E. Richard Stiehm (1966). Immune globulin levels in colostrum and breast milk and serum from formula- and breast-fed newborns. *Proceedings of the Society for Experimental Biology and Medicine* **122**, 1098–1100.

Anaokar, Sunil G., and Philip L. Garry (1981). Effects of maternal iron nutrition during lactation on milk iron and rat neonatal iron status. *American Journal of Clinical Nutrition* **34**, 1505–1512.

Andersen, Anders Myboe, and Vibeke Schiøler (1982). Influence of breast-feeding patterns on pituitary-ovarian axis of women in an industrialized community. *American Journal of Obstetrics and Gynecology* **143**, 673–677.

Anderson, Peter (1983). The reproductive role of the human breast. *Current Anthropology* **24**:1, 25–45.

Aono, Toshihiro, Takenori Shioji, Tsuneo Shoda, and Keiichi Kurachi (1977). The initiation of human lactation and prolactin response to suckling. *Journal of Clinical Endocrinology and Metabolism* **44**, 1101-1106.

Arena, Jay M. (1980). Drugs and chemicals excreted in breast milk. *Pediatric Annals* **9**, 452–457.

Arman, Pamela (1979). Milk from semi-domesticated ruminants. *World Review of Nutrition and Dietetics* **33**, 198–227.

Arnold, Roland R., Jiri Mestecky, and Jerry R. McGhee (1976). Naturally occurring secretory immunoglobulin A antibodies to Streptococcus mutans in human colostrum and saliva. *Infection and Immunity* **14**, 355–362.

Arroyave, Guillermo (1976). Nutrition in pregnancy. Studies in Central America and Panama. *Archivos Latinoamericanos de Nutrición* **26**, 129–157.

Arroyave, Guillermo, Ivan Beghin, Marina Flores, Cecelia Soto de Guido, and Jose Mariá Ticas (1974). Efectos del consumo de azúcar fortificada con retinol por la madre embarazada y lactante cuya dieta habitual es baja en vitamina A. Estudio de la madre y del ninõ. *Archivos Latinoamericanos de Nutrición* **24**, 485–512.

Asantila, Tuula, Tapani Sovari, Toivo Hirvonen, and Paavo Toivanen (1973). Xenogenic reactivity of human fetal lymphocytes. *Journal of Immunology* **111**, 984–987.

Asher, Patria (1952). The incidence and significance of breast feeding in infants admitted to hospital. *Archives of the Diseases of Childhood* **27**, 270–272.

Atkinson, S. A., M. H. Bryan, and G. H. Anderson (1978). Human milk: Difference in nitrogen concentration in milk from mothers of term and premature infants. *Journal of Pediatrics* **93**, 67–69.

Atkinson, S. A., I. C. Radde, G. W. Chance, M. H. Bryan, and G. H. Anderson (1980). Macro-mineral content of milk obtained during early lactation from mothers of premature infants. *Early Human Development* **4**, 5–14.

Austin, James E. (1978). The perilous journey of nutrition evaluation. *American Journal of Clinical Nutrition* **31**, 2324–2338.

Bachrach, Steven, Julian Fisher, and John S. Parks (1979). An outbreak of vitamin D deficiency rickets in a susceptible population. *Pediatrics* **64**, 871–877.

Badraoui, M. Hamdi H., and Fouad I. Hefnawi (1979). Ovarian function during lactation. In *Human Reproductive Medicine*. Vol. 3. *Human Ovulation: Mechanisms, Prediction, Detection and Induction*, edited by E. S. E. Hafez. North-Holland, Amsterdam, pp. 233–241.

Baird, David T., Alan S. McNeilly, Robert S. Sawers, and Richard M. Sharpe (1979). Failure of estrogen-induced discharge of luteinizing hormone in lactating women. *Journal of Clinical Endocrinology and Metabolism* **49**, 500–506.

Ballard, Jeanne L., Kathy Kazmaier Novak, and Marshall Driver (1979). A simplified score for assessment of fetal maturation of newly born infants. *Journal of Pediatrics* **95**, 769–774.

Barr, D. G. D., D. H. Schmerling, and A. Prader (1972). Catch-up growth in malnutrition, studied in celiac disease after institution of gluten-free diet. *Pediatric Research* **6**, 521–527.

Barrell, R. A. E., and Michael G. M. Rowland (1980). Commercial milk products and indigenous weaning foods in a rural West African environment: A bacteriological perspective. *Journal of Hygiene* **84**, 191–202.

Bates, Christopher J., Andrew M. Prentice, Ann Prentice, W. H. Lamb, and Roger G.

Whitehead (1983). The effect of vitamin C supplementation on lactating women in Keneba, a West African rural community. *International Journal for Vitamin and Nutrition Research* **53**, 68–76.

Bates, Christopher J., Andrew M. Prentice, Alison A. Paul, Barbara A. Sutcliffe, Michael Watkinson, and Roger G. Whitehead (1981). Riboflavin status in Gambian pregnant and lactating women and its implications for recommended dietary allowances. *American Journal of Clinical Nutrition* **34**, 928–935.

Bates, Christopher J., Andrew M. Prentice, Ann Prentice, Alison A. Paul, and Roger G. Whitehead (1982). Seasonal variations in ascorbic acid status and breast milk ascorbic acid levels in rural Gambian women in relation to dietary intake. *Transactions of the Royal Society of Tropical Medicine and Hygiene* **76**, 341–347.

Battaglia, Frederick C., and Michael A. Simmons (1978). The low-birth-weight infant. In *Human Growth*. Vol. 2. *Postnatal Growth*, edited by Frank Falkner and James M. Tanner. Plenum, New York, pp. 507–555.

Bazaral, Michael, H. Alice Orgel, and Robert N. Hamburger (1971). IgE levels in normal infants and mothers and an inheritance hypothesis. *Journal of Immunology* **107**, 794–801.

Beasley, R. Palmer, Cladd E. Stevens, I-Sen Shiao, and Hsien-Chieh Meng (1975). Evidence against breast feeding as a mechanism for vertical transmission of Hepatitis B. *The Lancet* **2**(18 Oct.), 740–741.

Beaton, George H. (1979). Nutritional needs of the pregnant and lactating mother. In *The Mother/Child Dyad—Nutritional Aspects*. Symposia of the Swedish Nutrition Foundation, XIV, edited by Leif Hambraeus and Stig Sjölin. Almqvist and Wiksell International, Stockholm, pp. 26–34.

Beer, Alan E., and Rupert E. Billingham (1975). Immunologic benefits and hazards of milk in maternal-perinatal relationship. *Annals of Internal Medicine* **83**, 865–871.

Beerens, Henri, C. Romond, and C. Neut (1980). Influence of breast-feeding on bifid flora of the newborn intestine. *American Journal of Clinical Nutrition* **33**, 2434–2439.

Beisel, William R., Robert Edelman, Kathleen Nauss, and Robert M. Suskind (1981). Single-nutrient effects on immunologic functions. Report of a workshop sponsored by the Department of Food and Nutrition and its advisory group of the American Medical Association. *Journal of the American Medical Association* **245**, 53–58.

Belavady, Bhavani (1980). Dietary supplementation and improvements in the lactation performance of Indian women. In *Maternal Nutrition during Pregnancy and Lactation. A Nestlé Workshop*. Lutry/Lausanne: April 26th and 27th 1969, edited by Hugo Aebi and Roger G. Whitehead. Nestlé Foundation Publication Series no. 1. Hans Huber, Bern, pp. 264–273.

Belavady, Bhavani, and C. Gopalan (1959). Chemical composition of human milk in poor Indian women. *Indian Journal of Medical Research* **47**, 234–245.

Bellanti, Joseph A. (1985). *Immunology. Basic Processes*. 2d ed. Saunders, Philadelphia.

Bellanti, Joseph A., and Josef V. Kadlec (1985). General immunobiology. In *Immunology III*, edited by Joseph A. Bellanti. Saunders, Philadelphia, pp. 16–53.

Bellanti, Joseph A., Lata S. Nerurkar, and Barbara J. Zeligs (1979). Host defenses in the fetus and neonate: Studies of the alveolar macrophage during maturation. *Pediatrics* **64**(suppl.), 726–739.

Benacerraf, Baruj, and Emil R. Unanue (1979). *Textbook of Immunology*. Williams & Wilkins, Baltimore.

Berger, Rosemarie, F. Hadziselimovic, M. Just, and P. Reigel (1983). Effect of feeding human milk on nosocomial rotavirus infections in an infants ward. *Developments in Biological Standardization* **53**, 219–228.

Berio, Ann-Jacqueline (1984). The analysis of time allocation and activity patterns in nutrition and rural development planning. *Food and Nutrition Bulletin* **6** (1), 53–68.

Berman, Michael L., Kenneth Hanson, and Ida L. Hellman (1972). Effect of breast-feeding on postpartum menstruation, ovulation, and pregnancy in Alaskan Eskimos. *American Journal of Obstetrics and Gynecology* **114**, 524–534.

Bhaskaram, C., N. Raghuramulu, and Vinodini Reddy (1977). Cell-mediated immunity and immunoglobulin levels in light-for-date infants. *Acta Paediatrica Scandinavica* **66**, 617–619.

Billewicz, W. Z., H. M. Fellowes, and C. A. Hytten (1976). Comments on the critical metabolic mass and the age of menarche. *Annals of Human Biology* **3**, 51–59.

Blanc, Bernard (1981). Biochemical aspects of human milk—Comparison with bovine milk. *World Review of Nutrition and Dietetics* **36**, 1–89.

Boackel, Robert J., Kenneth M. Pruitt, and Jiri Mestecky (1974). The interactions of human complement with interfacially aggregated preparations of human secretory IgA. *Immunochemistry* **11**, 543–548.

Boldman, Rosanne, and Dwayne M. Reed (1976). Worldwide variations in low birth weight. In *The Epidemiology of Prematurity*. Proceedings of a working conference held at NICHD/NIH, Bethesda, Maryland, November 8–9, 1976, edited by Dwayne M. Reed and Fiona J. Stanley. Urban & Schwarzenberg, Baltimore, pp. 39–51.

Bongaarts, John P. (1980). Does malnutrition affect fecundity: A summary of evidence. *Science* **208**(9 May), 564–569.

Bongaarts, John P. (1984). The proximate determinants of natural marital fertility. In *Determinants of Fertility in Developing Countries*. Vol. 1., edited by Rodolfo A. Bulatao and Ronald D. Lee with Paula E. Hollerbach and John P. Bongaarts. Academic Press, New York, pp. 132–138.

Bongaarts, John P., and Hernán Delgado (1979). Effects of nutritional status on fertility in rural Guatemala. In *Natural Fertility Patterns and Determinants of Natural Fertility: Proceedings of a Seminar on Natural Fertility*, edited by Henri Leridon and Jane A. Menken. Ordina Editions, Liège, Belgium, pp. 107–133.

Bonnar, J., M. Franklin, P. N. Nott, and Alan S. McNeilly (1975). Effect of breast-feeding on pituitary-ovarian function after childbirth. *British Medical Journal* **4**, 82–84.

Brandt, Ingeborg (1978). Growth dynamics of low-birth-weight infants with emphasis on the perinatal period. In *Human Growth*. Vol. 2. *Postnatal Growth*, edited by Frank Falkner and James M. Tanner. Plenum, New York, pp. 557–617.

Brasel, Jo Anne (1978). Impact of malnutrition on reproductive endocrinology. *Nutrition and Human Reproduction*, edited by W. Henry Mosley. Plenum, New York, pp. 29–60.

Bravo, Ilse López, Carmen Cabiol, Sara Arcuch, Eliana Rivera, and Sergio Vargas (1984). Breast-feeding, weight gains, diarrhea, and malnutrition in the first year of life. *Bulletin of the Pan American Health Organization* **18**, 151–163.

Brazleton, T. Berry (1977). Implications of infant development among the Mayan Indians of Mexico. In *Culture and Infancy: Variations in the Human Experience*, edited by P. Herbert Leiderman, Steven R. Tulkin, and Anne Rosenfeld. The Child Psychology Series. Academic Press, New York, pp. 151–187.

Briscoe, John (1979). The quantitative effect of infection on the use of food by young children in poor countries. *American Journal of Clinical Nutrition* **32**, 648–676.

Brown, Kenneth H., Robert E. Black, A. D. Robertson, and Stan Becker (1983). Effects of season and illness on the dietary intake of weanlings during longitudinal studies in rural Bangladesh. Department of International Health, Johns Hopkins University, Baltimore.

Brown, Roy E. (1978). Weaning foods in developing countries. *American Journal of Clinical Nutrition* **31**, 2066–2072.

Bullen, J. J., Henry J. Rogers, and E. Griffith (1978). Nutrient deficiencies in breast-fed infants. *New England Journal of Medicine* **299**(28 Dec.), 1471.

Bullen, J. J., Henry J. Rogers, and L. Leigh (1972). Iron-binding proteins in milk and resistance to *Escherichia coli* infection in infants. *British Medical Journal* **1**(8 Jan.), 69–75.

Butler, J. E. (1979). Immunologic aspects of breast feeding, antiinfectious activity of breast milk. *Seminars in Perinatology* **3**, 255–270.

Butte, Nancy F., Cutberto Garza, E. O'Brian Smith, and Buford L. Nichols (1983). Evaluation of the deuterium dilution technique against the test-weighting procedure for the determination of breast milk intake. *American Journal of Clinical Nutrition* **37**, 996–1003.

Butte, Nancy F., Cutberto Garza, Janice E. Stuff, E. O'Brian Smith, and Buford L. Nichols (1984a). Effect of maternal diet and body composition on lactational performance. *American Journal of Clinical Nutrition* **39**, 296–306.

Butte, Nancy F., Randall M. Goldblum, L. M. Fehl, K. Loftin, E. O'Brian Smith, Cutberto Garza, and Armond S. Goldman (1984b). Daily ingestion of immunologic components in human milk during the first four months of life. *Acta Paediatrica Scandinavica* **73**, 296–301.

Butz, William P., Jean-Pierre Habicht, and Julie DaVanzo (1984). Environmental factors in the relationship between breastfeeding and infant mortality: The role of sanitation and water in Malaysia. *American Journal of Epidemiology* **119**, 516–525.

Caldwell, John C., and Pat Caldwell (1977). The role of marital sexual abstinence in determining fertility: A study of the Yoruba in Nigeria. *Population Studies* **31**, 193–217.

Cameron, N. (1976). Weight and skinfold variation at menarche and the critical body weight hypothesis. *Annals of Human Biology* **3**, 279–282.

Canadian Paediatric Society, Nutrition Committee (1981). Feeding the low-birthweight infant. *Canadian Medical Association Journal* **124**, 1301–1311.

Caräel, Michel (1978). Relations between birth intervals and nutrition in three Central African populations (Zaire). In *Nutrition and Human Reproduction*, edited by W. Henry Mosley. Plenum, New York, pp. 365–384.

Casey, Clare E., Philip A. Walravens, and K. Michael Hambidge (1981). Availability of zinc: Loading tests with human milk, cow's milk and infant formulas. *Pediatrics* **68**, 394–396.

Chandra, R. K. (1979). Prospective studies of the effect of breast feeding on incidence of infection and allergy. *Acta Paediatrica Scandinavica* **68**, 691–694.

Chandra, R. K. (1981). Breast feeding, growth and morbidity. *Nutrition Research* **1**, 25–31.

Chandra, R. K. (1982). Physical growth of exclusively breast-fed infants. *Nutrition Research* **2**, 275–276.

Chávez, Adolfo, and Celia Martínez (1973). Nutrition and development of infants from poor rural areas. III. Maternal nutrition and its consequences on fertility. *Nutrition Reports International* **7**, 1–8.

Chávez, Adolfo, and Celia Martínez (1980). Effects of maternal undernutrition and dietary supplementation on milk production. In *Maternal Nutrition during Pregnancy and Lactation: A Nestlé Workshop*. Lutry/Lausanne, April 26th and 27th 1969, edited by Hugo Aebi and Roger G. Whitehead. Nestlé Foundation Publication Series no. 1. Hans Huber, Bern, pp. 274–284.

Chen, Lincoln C., Shamsa Ahmed, Melita C. Gesche, and W. Henry Mosley (1974). A prospective study of birth interval dynamics in rural Bangladesh. *Population Studies* **28**, 277–297.

Chen, Lincoln C., A. K. M. Alauddin Chowdhury, and Sandra L. Huffman (1979). Seasonal dimensions of energy protein malnutrition in rural Bangladesh: The role of agriculture, dietary practices, and infection. *Ecology of Food and Nutrition* **8**, 175–187.

Chowdhury, A. K. M. Alauddin (1978). Effect of maternal nutrition on fertility in rural Bangladesh. In *Nutrition and Human Reproduction*, edited by W. Henry Mosley. Plenum, New York, pp. 401–410.

Christakis, George, ed. (1973). *Nutritional Assessment in Health Programs*. American Public

Cohen, Irun R., and Leslie C. Norins (1968). Antibodies of the IgG, IgM, and IgA classes in newborn and adult sera reactive with gram-negative bacteria. *Journal of Clinical Investigation* **47**, 1053–1062.

Corsini, Carlo A. (1979). Is the fertility-reducing effect of lactation really substantial? In *Natural Fertility: Patterns and Determinants of Natural Fertility: Proceedings of a Seminar on Natural Fertility*, edited by Henri Leridon and Jane A. Menken. Ordina Editions, Liège, Belgium (for the International Union for the Scientific Study of Population), pp. 195–215.

Coward, W. A., T. J. Cole, M. B. Sawyer, and Andrew M. Prentice (1982). Breast-milk intake measurement in mixed-fed infants by administration of deuterium oxide to their mothers. *Human Nutrition: Clinical Nutrition* **36C**, 141–148.

Coward, W. A., Alison A. Paul, and Andrew M. Prentice (1984). The impact of malnutrition on human lactation: Observations from community studies. *Federation Proceedings* **43**, 2432–2437.

Coward, W. A., M. B. Sawyer, Roger G. Whitehead, Andrew M. Prentice, and Janet Evans (1979). New method for measuring milk intakes in breast-fed babies. *The Lancet* **2**(7 July), 13–14.

CPS. See Canadian Paediatric Society.

Craft, I. L., D. M. Matthews, and J. C. Linnell (1971). Cobalamins in human pregnancy and lactation. *Journal of Clinical Pathology* **24**, 449–455.

Cravioto, Joaquín (1972). The ecologic approach to the study of nutrition and mental development: The Mexico study. In *Nutrition, Growth and Development of North American Indian Children*, edited by William M. Moore, Marjorie M. Silverberg, and Merrill S. Read. DHEW Publication no. (NIH) 72–76. National Institutes of Health, Public Health Service, U.S. Department of Health, Education, and Welfare [Bethesda, Md.], pp. 169–184.

Cravioto, Joaquín, and Elsa R. DeLicardie (1976). Microenvironmental factors in severe protein-calorie malnutrition. In *Nutrition and Agricultural Development. Significance of Potential for the Tropics*, edited by Nevin S. Scrimshaw and Moisés Béhar. Plenum, New York, pp. 25–35.

Crisol, M., and James F. Phillips (1975). Lactation and amenorrhea life tables from the 1974 National Acceptor Survey. Research Note no. 34, Population Institute, University of the Philippines System, [Manila].

Cunningham, Allan S. (1977). Morbidity in breast-fed and artificially fed infants. *Journal of Pediatrics* **90**, 726–729.

Cunningham, Allan S. (1979). Morbidity in breast-fed and artificially fed infants. II. *Journal of Pediatrics* **95**, 685–689.

Cunningham, Allan S. (1981). Breast-feeding and morbidity in industrialized countries: An update. In *Advances in International Maternal and Child Health*. Vol. 1., edited by Derrick B. Jelliffe and E. F. Patrice Jelliffe. Oxford Medical Publications. Oxford University Press, Oxford, pp. 128–168.

Cuthbertson, W. F. J. (1976). Essential fatty acid requirements in infancy. *American Journal of Clinical Nutrition* **29**, 559–568.

Cushing, Alice H., and Linda Anderson (1982). Diarrhea in breast-fed and non-breast-fed infants. *Pediatrics* **70**, 921–925.

Dagan, R., and H. Pridan (1982). Relationship of breast feeding versus bottle feeding with emergency room visits and hospitalization for infectious diseases. *European Journal of Pediatrics* **139**, 192–194.

Dale, G., Monica E. Goldfinch, J. R. Sibert, and J. K. G. Webb (1975). Plasma osmolality, sodium, and urea in healthy breast-fed and bottle-fed infants in Newcastle upon Tyne. *Archives of Disease in Childhood* **50**, 731–734.

DaVanzo, Julie, and J. Haaga (1982). Anatomy of a fertility decline: Peninsular Malaysia,

1950–1976. *Population Studies* **36**, 373–393.

Davies, D. P. (1979). Is inadequate breast-feeding an important cause of failure to thrive? *Lancet* **1** (10 March), 541–542.

Davies, D. P., and R. Saunders (1973). Blood urea: Normal values in early infancy related to feeding practices. *Archives of Disease in Childhood* **48**, 563–565.

Davis, William H. (1913). Statistical comparison of the mortality of breast-fed and bottle-fed infants. *American Journal of Diseases of Children* **5**, 234–247.

de Château, P., Hertha Holmberg, Kerstin Jakobsson, and Jan Winberg (1977). A study of factors promoting and inhibiting lactation. *Developmental Medicine and Child Neurology* **19**, 575–584.

Deeny, James, and Eric T. Murdock (1944). Infant feeding in relation to mortality in the city of Belfast. *British Medical Journal* **1**(29 Jan.), 146–148.

Delgado, Hernán L., Elena Hurtado, Victor Valverde, and Robert E. Klein (1981). Lactation in rural Guatemala: Nutritional effects on the mother and the infant. Division of Human Development, Institute of Nutrition of Central America and Panama, Guatemala City.

Delgado, Hernán L., Aaron Lechtig, Reynaldo Martorell, Elena Brineman, and Robert E. Klein (1978). Nutrition, lactation, and postpartum amenorrhea. *American Journal of Clinical Nutrition* **31**, 322–327.

DelPinal, Jorge H. (1981). Breastfeeding and infant mortality in Guatemala. Paper presented at the annual meeting of the Population Association of America, Washington, D.C., 26–28 March.

Delvoye, Pierre, J. Delogne-Desnoeck, and Claude Robyn (1976). Serum-prolactin in long-lasting lactation amenorrhoea. *The Lancet* **2**(7 Aug.), 288–289.

Delvoye, Pierre, J. Delogne-Desnoeck, and Claude Robyn (1980). Hyperprolactinaemia during prolonged lactation: Evidence for anovulatory cycles and inadequate corpus luteum. *Clinical Endocrinology* **13**, 243–247.

Delvoye, Pierre, M. Demaegd, J. Delogne-Desnoeck, and Claude Robyn (1977). The influence of the frequency of nursing and of previous lactation experiences on serum prolactin in lactating mothers. *Journal of Biosocial Science* **9**, 447–451.

D'Souza, S. W., and Patricia Black (1979). A study of infant growth in relation to the type of feeding. *Early Human Development* **3**, 245–255.

de Swiet, Michael, Peter Fayers, and Lesley Cooper (1977). Effect of feeding habit on weight in infancy. *The Lancet* **1**(23 Apr.), 892–894.

Devadas, Rajammal P., and N. Mangalam (1970). The nutritional status of nursing mothers in a village. *Indian Journal of Nutrition and Dietetics* **7**, 153–159.

Devadas, Rajammal P., J. R. Baby Anuradha, and B. Sharadambal (1971). Evaluation of an applied nutrition feeding programme on the nutritional status of nursing women. *Indian Journal of Nutrition and Dietetics* **8**, 143–148.

Devadas, Rajammal P., P. Vijayalakshmi, and P. Nagalakshmi (1978). Nutritional profile of selected nursing mothers in Coimbatore City. *Indian Journal of Nutrition and Dietetics* **15**, 367–370.

Dewey, Kathryn G., Dorothy A. Finley, and Bo Lönnerdal (1984). Breast milk volume and composition during late lactation (7–20 months). *Journal of Pediatric Gastroenterology and Nutrition* **3**, 713–720.

Diaz-Jouanen, Efrain P., and Ralph C. Williams (1974). T and B lymphocytes in human colostrum. *Clinical Immunology and Immunopathology* **3**, 248–255.

Dine, Mark S., Peter S. Gartside, Charles J. Glueck, Larry Rheines, Gail Greene, and Philip Khoury (1979). Where do the heaviest children come from? A prospective study of white children from birth to 5 years of age. *Pediatrics* **63**, 1–7.

Dixon, Frank J., David W. Talmage, Paul H. Maurer, and Maria Deichmiller (1952). The half-life of homologous gamma globulin (antibody) in several species. *Journal of*

Experimental Medicine **96**, 313–318.

Dolby, Jean M., and Susan Stephens (1983). Antibodies to *Escherichia coli* O antigens and the in-vitro bacteriostatic properties of human milk and its IgA. *Acta Paediatrica Scandinavica* **72**, 577–582.

Dossett, John H., Ralph C. Williams, and Paul G. Quie (1969). Studies on interaction of bacteria, serum factors and polymorphonuclear leukocytes in mothers and newborns. *Pediatrics* **44**, 49–57.

Douglas, J. W. B. (1950). The extent of breast feeding in Great Britain in 1946, with special reference to the health and survival of children. *Journal of Obstetrics and Gynaecology of the British Empire* **57**, 335–361.

Downham, M. A. P. S., R. Scott, D. G. Sims, J. K. G. Webb, and P. S. Gardner (1976). Breast-feeding protects against respiratory syncytial virus infections. *British Medical Journal* **2**(31 July), 274–276.

Drew, P. A., O. M. Petrucco, and D. J. C. Shearman (1983). Inhibition by colostrum of the responses of peripheral blood mononuclear cells to mitogens. *Australian Journal of Experimental Biology and Medical Science* **61**, 451–460.

Drew, P. A., O. M. Petrucco, and D. J. C. Shearman (1984). A factor present in human milk, but not colostrum, which is cytotoxic for human lymphocytes. *Clinical and Experimental Immunology* **55**, 437–443.

Dubois, Sheila, Donald E. Hill, and George H. Beaton (1979). An examination of factors believed to be associated with infantile obesity. *American Journal of Clinical Nutrition* **32**, 1997–2004.

Dubowitz, Lilly M. S., Victor Dubowitz, and Cissie Goldberg (1970). Clinical assessment of gestational age in the newborn infant. *Journal of Pediatrics* **77**, 1–10.

Duchen, M. R., and Alan S. McNeilly (1980). Hyperprolactinaemia and long-term lactational amenorrhoea. *Clinical Endocrinology* **12**, 621–627.

Dugdale, A. E. (1971). The effect of the type of feeding on weight gain and illness in infants. *British Journal of Nutrition* **26**, 423–432.

Dugdale, A. E. (1980). Infant feeding, growth and mortality: A 20-year study of an Australian aboriginal community. *Medical Journal of Australia* **2**, 380–385.

Duncan, John R., and Lucille S. Hurley (1978). Intestinal absorption of zinc: A role for a zinc-binding ligand in milk. *American Journal of Physiology* **235**, E556–559.

Durnin, John Valentine George Andrew (1980). Food consumption and energy balance during pregnancy and lactation in New Guinea. In *Maternal Nutrition during Pregnancy and Lactation: A Nestlé Foundation Workshop*, Lutry/Lausanne, April 26–27, 1979, edited by Hugo Aebi and Roger G. Whitehead. Nestlé Foundation Publication Series no. 1. Hans Huber, Bern, Switzerland, pp. 86–95.

Eastman, Nicholson J., and Esther Jackson (1968). Weight relationships in pregnancy. I. The bearing of maternal weight gain and pre-pregnancy weight on birth weight in full term pregnancies. *Obstetrical and Gynecological Survey* **23**, 1003–1025.

Edidin, Deborah V., Lynne L. Levitsky, William Schey, Nives Dumbovic, and Alfonso Campos (1980). Resurgence of nutritional rickets associated with breast-feeding and special dietary practices. *Pediatrics* **65**, 232–235.

Edozien, Joseph C. (1979). Dietary influences on human lactation performance. In *Maternal Nutrition during Pregnancy and Lactation: A Nestlé Foundation Workshop*, Lutry/Lausanne, April 26–27, 1979, edited by Hugo Aebi and Roger G. Whitehead. Nestlé Foundation Publication Series no. 1. Hans Huber, Bern, Switzerland, pp. 203–221.

Eggert, F. Michael, and B. W. Gurner (1984). Reaction of human colostral and early milk antibodies with oral *Streptococci*. *Infection and Immunity* **44**, 660–664.

Elandt-Johnson, Regina C., and Norman L. Johnson (1980). *Survival Models and Data Analysis*. Wiley Series in Probability and Mathematical Statistics: Applied Probability and Statistics. Wiley, New York.

Emery, John L., P. G. F. Swift, and E. Worthy (1974). Hypernatraemia and uraemia in unexpected death in infancy. *Archives of Disease in Childhood* **49**, 686–692.

Ernst, Judith A., Ralph J. Wynn, and Richard L. Schreiner (1981). Starvation with hypernatremic dehydration in two breast-fed infants. *Journal of the American Dietetic Association* **79**, 126–130.

Evans, D. G., and J. W. G. Smith (1963). Response of the young infant to active immunization. *British Medical Bulletin* **19**, 225–229.

Fallot, Mary E., John L. Boyd, III, and Frank A. Oski (1980). Breast-feeding reduces incidence of hospital admissions for infection in infants. *Pediatrics* **65**, 1121–1124.

Fållström, S. P., S. Ahlstedt, B. Carlsson, B. Wettergren, and L. Å. Hanson (1984). Influence of breast feeding on the development of cow's milk protein antibodies and the IgE level. *International Archives of Allergy and Applied Immunology* **75**, 87–91.

Feachem, R. G., and M. A. Koblinsky (1984). Interventions for the control of diarrhoeal diseases among young children: Promotion of breast-feeding. *Bulletin of the World Health Organization* **62**, 271–291.

Fenuku, R. I. A., and S. N. Earl-Quarcoo (1978). Serum calcium, magnesium and inorganic phosphate during lactation. *Tropical and Geographical Medicine* **30**, 495–498.

Ferguson, Anne, and Stephan Strobel (1984). Potential effects of weaning on intestinal immunity. Unpublished manuscript. Gastro-Intestinal Unit, Western General Hospital, Edinburgh, and University of Edinburgh, Scotland.

Fergusson, David M., L. John Horwood, Frederick T. Shannon, and Brent Taylor (1978). Infant health and breast-feeding during the first 16 weeks of life. *Australian Paediatric Journal* **14**, 254–258.

Fergusson, David M., L. John Horwood, Frederick T. Shannon, and Brent Taylor (1981). Breast-feeding, gastrointestinal and lower respiratory illness in the first two years. *Australian Paediatric Journal* **17**, 191–195.

Ferris, Ann G., Mary J. Laus, David W. Hosmer, and Virginia A. Beal (1980). The effect of diet on weight gain in infancy. *American Journal of Clinical Nutrition* **33**, 2635–2642.

Ferry, Benoit (1981). *Breastfeeding.* World Fertility Survey Comparative Studies, Cross National Summaries, no. 13. International Statistical Institute, Voorburg, Netherlands.

Fleisher, Thomas A., John R. Luckasen, Andrej Sabada, Richard C. Gehrtz, and John H. Kersey (1975). T and B lymphocyte subpopulations in children. *Pediatrics* **55**, 162–165.

Fomon, Samuel J. (1967). Body composition of the male reference infant during the first year of life. *Pediatrics* **40**, 863–870.

Fomon, Samuel J. (1974). *Infant Nutrition.* 2d ed. Saunders, Philadelphia.

Fomon, Samuel J., and Charles D. May (1958). Metabolic studies of normal full-term infants fed pasteurized human milk. *Pediatrics* **22**, 101–115.

Fomon, Samuel J., and Ronald G. Strauss (1978). Nutrient deficiencies in breast-fed infants. *New England Journal of Medicine* **299**(28 Dec.), 1471.

Fomon, Samuel J., Ekhard E. Ziegler, and Héctor D. Vázquez (1977). Human milk and the small premature infant. *American Journal of Disease of Children* **131**, 463–467.

Ford, J. E., B. A. Law, Valerie M. E. Marshall, and B. Reiter (1977). Influence of the heat treatment of human milk on some of its protective constituents. *Journal of Pediatrics* **90**, 29–35.

Ford, J. E., K. J. Scott, B. F. Sansom, and P. J. Taylor (1975). Some observations on the possible nutritional significance of vitamin B_{12} and folate-binding proteins in milk. Absorption of [^{58}Co]cyanocobalamin by suckling piglets. *British Journal of Nutrition* **34**, 469–492.

Forman, M. R., B. I. Graubard, H. J. Hoffman, R. Beren, E. E. Harley, and P. Bennett (1984). The Pima infant feeding study: Breast feeding and gastroenteritis in the first year of life. *American Journal of Epidemiology* **119**, 335–349.

France, Gene L., Daniel J. Marmer, and Russell W. Steele (1980). Breast-feeding and Salmonella infection. *American Journal of Diseases of Children* **134**, 147–152.

Frank, Arthur L., Larry H. Taber, W. P. Glezen, Gary L. Kasel, Cristine R. Wells, and Abel Paredes (1982). Breast-feeding and respiratory virus infection. *Pediatrics* **70**, 239–245.

French, Jean G. (1967). Relationship of morbidity to the feeding patterns of Navajo children from birth through twenty-four months. *American Journal of Clinical Nutrition* **20**, 375–385.

Friedman, Glenn, and Stanley J. Goldberg (1975). Concurrent and subsequent serum cholesterol of breast- and formula-fed infants. *American Journal of Clinical Nutrition* **28**, 42–45.

Frisch, Rose E. (1975). Demographic implications of the biological determinants of female fecundity. *Social Biology* **22**, 17–22.

Frisch, Rose E. (1978). Population, food intake, and fertility. *Science* **199**(6 Jan.), 22–30.

Fudenberg, H. Hugh, Daniel P. Stites, Joseph L. Caldwell, and Vivian J. Wells (1980). *Basic and Clinical Immunology*. 3d ed. Lang Medical, Los Altos, Calif.

Garrow, J. S., and M. C. Pike (1967). The long-term prognosis of severe infantile malnutrition. *The Lancet* **1**(7 Jan.), 1–4.

Garry, Philip J., George M. Owen, Elizabeth M. Hooper, and Barbara A. Gilbert (1981). Iron absorption from human milk and formula with and without iron supplementation. *Pediatric Research* **15**, 822–828.

Geissler, Catherine, Doris H. Calloway, and S. Margen (1978). Lactation and pregnancy in Iran. II. Diet and nutritional status. *American Journal of Clinical Nutrition* **31**, 341–354.

Gerrard, John W., and Mehdi Shenassa (1983a). Food allergy: Two common types as seen in breast and formula fed babies. *Annals of Allergy* **50**, 375–379.

Gerrard, John W., and Mehdi Shenassa (1983b). Sensitization to substances in breast milk: Recognition, management and significance. *Annals of Allergy* **51**, 300–302.

Ginsburg, Bengt-Erik, and Rolf Zetterström (1980). Serum cholesterol concentrations in early infancy. *Acta Paediatrica Scandinavica* **69**, 581–585.

Gitlin, David, and Anita Biasucci (1969). Development of γG, γA, γM, B/1C, B/1A, C'^1 esterase inhibitor, ceruloplasmin, transferrin, hemopexin, haptoglobin, fibrinogen, plasminogen, α1-antitrypsin, orosomucoid, B-lipoprotein, α2-macroglobulin, and prealbumin in the human conceptus. *Journal of Clinical Investigation* **48**, 1433–1446.

Gitlin, David, Jesús Kumate, Juan Urrusti, and Carlos Morales (1964). The selectivity of the human placenta in the transfer of plasma proteins from mother to fetus. *Journal of Clinical Investigation* **43**, 1938–1951.

Gitlin, David, Fred S. Rosen, and J. Gabriel Michael (1963). Transient 19S gamma$_1$-globulin deficiency in the newborn infant and its significance. *Pediatrics* **31**, 197–208.

Glasier, Anna, Alan S. McNeilly, and Peter W. Howie (1983). Fertility after childbirth: Changes in serum gonadotrophin levels in bottle and breast feeding women. *Clinical Endocrinology* **19**, 493–501.

Glass, Roger I., Ann-Mari Svennerholm, Barbara J. Stoll, M. R. Khan, K. M. Belayet Hossain, M. Imdadul Huq, and Jan Holmgren (1983). Protection against cholera in breast-fed children by antibodies in breast milk. *New England Journal of Medicine* **308**(9 June), 1389–1392.

Goldberg, H. I., W. Rodrigues, A. M. T. Thome, Barbara Janowitz, and L. Morris (1984). Infant mortality and breast-feeding in north-eastern Brazil. *Population Studies* **38**, 105–115.

Goldman, Armond S., and C. Wayne Smith (1973). Host resistance factors in human milk. *Journal of Pediatrics* **82**, 1082–1090.

Goldman, Noreen, Charles F. Westoff, and Lois E. Paul (1985). Estimation of natural fertility from survey data, for second and higher order birth intervals: A summary of results.

Paper presented at the annual meeting of the Population Association of America, Boston, 28–30 March.

Goodhart, Robert S., and Maurice E. Shils, eds. (1980). *Modern Nutrition in Health and Disease*. 6th ed. Lea & Febiger, Philadelphia.

Gopalan, C. (1958). Studies on lactation in poor Indian communities. *Journal of Tropical Pediatrics* **4**(3), 87–97.

Gopalan, C., and Bhavani Belavady (1961). Nutrition and lactation. *Federation Proceedings* **20**(suppl. 7), 177–184.

Gordon, John E., Ishwari D. Chitkara, and John B. Wyon (1963). Weanling diarrhea. *American Journal of the Medical Sciences* **245**, 345–377.

Gracey, Michael, Delys E. Stone, Suharjono, and Sunoto (1974). Isolation of Candida species from the gastrointestinal tract in malnourished children. *American Journal of Clinical Nutrition* **27**, 345–349.

Graham, George G., and Blanca T. Adrianzen (1972). Late "catch-up" growth after severe infantile malnutrition. *Johns Hopkins Medical Journal* **131**, 204–211.

Greiner, Theodore H., Stina Almroth, and Michael C. Latham (1979). *The Economic Value of Breastfeeding (with Results from Research Conducted in Ghana and the Ivory Coast)*. Cornell International Nutrition Monograph Series no. 6. Division of Nutritional Sciences, New York State College of Human Ecology, New York State College of Agriculture and Life Sciences, Statutory Colleges of the State University at Cornell University, Ithaca.

Gross, Barbara Anne (1981). The hormonal and ecological correlates of lactation infertility. *International Journal of Fertility* **26**, 209–218.

Gross, Barbara Anne, and Creswell J. Eastman (1979). Prolactin secretion during prolonged lactational amenorrhea. *Australia and New Zealand Journal of Obstetrics and Gynaecology* **19**, 95–99.

Gross, Barbara Anne, and Creswell J. Eastman (1983a). Effect of breast-feeding status on prolactin secretion and resumption of menstruation. *Medical Journal of Australia* **1**, 313–317.

Gross, Barbara Anne, and Creswell J. Eastman (1983b). Prolactin and the return to ovulation in breastfeeding women. Endocrine Unit, Department of Medicine, Westmead Centre, Westmead, New South Wales, Australia. Summary of paper presented at Research Seminar on Breastfeeding, Family Planning and the Return to Ovulation, Manila, Philippines, August 8–11.

Gross, Robert L., and Paul M. Newberne (1980). Role of nutrition in immunologic function. *Physiological Reviews* **60**, 188–302.

Gross, Steven J., Richard J. David, Linda Bauman, and R. M. Tomarelli (1980). Nutritional composition of milk produced by mothers delivering preterm. *Journal of Pediatrics* **96**, 641–644.

Grossman, Harvey, Eileen Duggan, Sarah McCamman, Eleanor Welchert, and Stanley Hellerstein (1980). The dietary chloride deficiency syndrome. *Pediatrics* **66**, 366–374.

Grulee, Clifford G., Heyworth N. Sanforth, and Paul H. Herron (1934). Breast and artificial feeding. Influence on morbidity and mortality of twenty thousand infants. *Journal of the American Medical Association* **103**, 735–741.

Gullberg, Ragnhild (1974). Possible influence of vitamin B_{12}-binding protein in milk on the intestinal flora in breast-fed infants. II. Contents of unsaturated B_{12}-binding protein in meconium and faeces from breast-fed and bottle-fed infants. *Scandinavian Journal of Gastroenterology* **9**, 287–292.

Gunn, Robert A., Ann M. Kimball, Robert A. Pollard, John C. Feeley, Samir R. Dutta, P. P. Matthew, Rifaat A. Mahmood, and Myron M. Levine (1979). Bottle feeding as a risk factor for cholera in infants. *The Lancet* **2**(6 Oct.), 730–732.

Gurwith, Marc, Wanda Wenman, Dorothy Hinde, Sheila Feltham, and Harry Greenberg

(1981). A prospective study of rotavirus in infants and young children. *Journal of Infectious Diseases* **144**, 218–224.

Gussler, Judith D., and Linda H. Breisemeister (1980). The insufficient milk syndrome: A biocultural explanation. *Medical Anthropology* **4**, 145–174.

György, Paul (1971). The uniqueness of human milk. Biochemical aspects. *American Journal of Clinical Nutrition* **24**, 970–975.

Habicht, Jean-Pierre, Julie DaVanzo, William P. Butz, and Linda Meyers (1985). The contraceptive role of breastfeeding. *Population Studies* **39**, 213–232.

Hall, Barbara (1975). Changing composition of human milk and early development of an appetite control. *The Lancet* **1**(5 Apr.), 779–781.

Hall, Barbara (1979). Uniformity of human milk. *American Journal of Clinical Nutrition* **32**, 304–312.

Halsey, John F., Craig S. Mitchell, and Sara J. McKenzie (1983). The origins of secretory IgA in milk: A shift during lactation from a serum origin to local synthesis in the mammary gland. *Annals of the New York Academy of Science* **409**, 452–459.

Hambidge, K. Michael, Philip A. Walravens, Clare E. Casey, Ronald M. Brown, and Connie Bender (1979). Plasma zinc concentrations of breast-fed infants. *Journal of Pediatrics* **94**, 607–608.

Hamilton, Sahni, Barry M. Popkin, and Deborah Spicer (1984). *Women and Nutrition in the Third World Countries*. Praeger Special Studies. Praeger Scientific. Bergin & Garvey, South Hadley, Mass.

Hamosh, Margit, K. N. Sivasubramanian, Carol Salzman-Mann, and Paul Hamosh (1978). Fat digestion in the stomach of premature infants I. Characteristics of lipase activity. *Journal of Pediatrics* **93**, 674–679.

Hanafy, M. M., M. R. A. Morsey, Y. Seddick, Y. A. Habib, and M. el Lozy (1972). Maternal nutrition and lactation performance. A study in urban Alexandria. *Journal of Tropical Pediatrics and Environmental Child Health* **18**, 187–191.

Hanson, L. Å., and J. Winberg (1972). Breast milk and defence against infection in the newborn. *Archives of Disease in Childhood* **47**, 845–848.

Hanson, L. Å., S. Ahlstedt, B. Carlsson, and S. P. Fållström (1977). Secretory IgA antibodies against cow's milk protein in human milk and their possible effect in mixed feeding. *International Archives of Allergy and Applied Immunology* **54**, 457–462.

Harrison, G. A., A. J. Boyce, C. M. Platt, and S. Serjeantson (1975). Body composition changes during lactation in a New Guinea population. *Annals of Human Biology* **2**, 395–398.

Head, Judith R., and Alan E. Beer (1978). The immunologic role of viable leukocytic cells in mammary exosecretions. In *Lactation. A Comprehensive Treatise*. Vol. 4. *The Mammary Gland/Human Lactation/Milk Synthesis*, edited by Bruce Larson. Academic Press, New York, pp. 337–364.

Hennart, Ph., and H. L. Vis (1980). Breast-feeding and post partum amenorrhoea in central Africa. I. Milk production in rural areas. *Journal of Tropical Pediatrics* **26**, 177–183.

Hennart, Ph., J. Delogne-Desnoeck, H. L. Vis, and Claude Robyn (1981). Serum levels of prolactin and milk production in women during a lactation period of thirty months *Clinical Endocrinology* **14**, 349–353.

Hill, P., and F. Wynder (1976). Diet and prolactin release. *The Lancet* **2**(9 Oct.), 806–807.

Hitchcock, Nancy E., Michael Gracey, and Elisabeth N. Owles (1981). Growth of healthy breast-fed infants in the first six months. *The Lancet* **2**(11 July), 64–65.

Hodgson, Patricia A., Ralph D. Ellefson, Lila R. Elveback, Lloyd E. Harris, Ralph A. Nelson, and William H. Weidman (1976). Comparison of serum cholesterol in children fed high, moderate, or low cholesterol milk diets during neonatal period. *Metabolism* **25**, 739–746.

Hodgson, S. V. (1978). Early infant feeding and weight gain. *Journal of the Royal College of General Practitioners* **28**, 280–281.

Holmgren, Jan, Ann-Mari Svennerholm, and M. Lindblad (1983). Receptor-like glycocompounds in human milk that inhibit classical and El Tor *Vibrio cholerae* cell adherence (hemagglutination). *Infection and Immunity* **30**, 147–154.

Howarth, William J. (1905). The influence of feeding on the mortality of infants. *The Lancet* **2**(22 July), 210–213.

Howell, Nancy (1979). *Demography of the Dobe !Kung. Population and Social Structure: Advances in Historical Demography.* Academic Press, New York.

Howie, Peter W., and Alan S. McNeilly (1982). Effect of breast-feeding patterns on human birth intervals. *Journal of Reproduction and Fertility* **65**, 545–557.

Howie, Peter W., Alan S. McNeilly, Mary J. Houston, A. Cook, and H. Boyle (1981). Effect of supplementary food on suckling patterns and ovarian activity during lactation. *British Medical Journal* **283**, 757–759.

Howie, Peter W., Alan S. McNeilly, Mary J. Houston, A. Cook, and H. Boyle (1982a). Fertility after childbirth: Infant feeding patterns, basal prolactin levels and post-partum ovulation. *Endocrinology* **17**, 315–322.

Howie, Peter W., Alan S. McNeilly, Mary J. Houston, A. Cook, and H. Boyle (1982b). Fertility after childbirth: Post-partum ovulation and menstruation in bottle and breast feeding mothers. *Clinical Endocrinology* **17**, 323–332.

Hoyle, Bruce, Mohammed Yunus, and Lincoln C. Chen (1980). Breast-feeding and food intake among children with acute diarrheal disease. *American Journal of Clinical Nutrition* **33**, 2365–2371.

Huffman, Sandra L., A. K. M. Alauddin Chowdhury, and W. Henry Mosley (1978). Postpartum amenorrhea: How is it affected by maternal nutritional status? *Science* **200**(9 June), 1155–1157.

Huffman, Sandra L., A. K. M. Alauddin Chowdhury, and Zenas M. Sykes (1980). Lactation and fertility in rural Bangledesh. *Population Studies* **34**, 337–347.

Huffman, Sandra L., Kathleen Ford, Hubert A. Allen, Jr., and Peter Streble (1985). Nutrition and fertility in Bangladesh: Breastfeeding and postpartum amenorrhea. Paper presented at the annual meeting of the Population Association of American, Boston, 28–30 March.

Hull, Valerie J. (1978). A study of birth interval dynamics in rural Java. In *Nutrition and Human Reproduction*, edited by W. Henry Mosley. Plenum, New York, pp. 433–459.

Hull, Valerie J. (1981). The effects of hormonal contraceptives on lactation: Current findings, methodological considerations and future priorities. In "Breastfeeding Program, Policy and Research Issues," edited by Edward C. Baer and Beverly Winikoff. *Studies in Family Planning* **12**, 134–155.

Hull, Valerie J. (1984). *Breast-feeding and fertility in Yogyakarta.* Monograph Series no. 5. Yogyakarta, Indonesia: Population Studies Center, Gadjah Mada University.

Hytten, Frank E. (1964). Nutritional aspects of foetal growth. In *Proceedings of the Sixth International Congress of Nutrition. Edinburgh, 9th to 15th August 1963*, edited by D. P. Cuthbertson, C. F. Mills, and R. Livingston Passmore. E. & S. Livingstone, Edinburgh, pp. 59–65.

Hytten, Frank E., and Isabella Leitch (1971). *The Physiology of Human Pregnancy.* 2d ed. Lippincott, Philadelphia.

Inglis, G. C., R. G. Sommerville, and D. B. L. McClelland (1978). Anti-rotavirus antibody in human colostrum. *The Lancet* **1**(11 Mar.), 559–560.

International Union for the Scientific Study of Population. Demographic Dictionary Committee (1985). *Multilingual Demographic Dictionary. English Section*, adapted by Etienne van der Walle from the French Section edited by Louis Henry. 2d ed. Ordina Editions, Liège, Belgium.

IUSSP. See International Union for the Scientific Study of Population.

Jagadeesan, V., and Vinodini Reddy (1978). Serum complement and lysozyme levels in light-for-date infants. *Indian Journal of Medical Research* **67**, 965–967.

Jain, Anrudh Kumar, Albert I. Hermalin, and Te-Hsiung Sun (1979). Lactation and natural fertility. In *Natural Fertility: Patterns and Determinants of Natural Fertility: Proceedings of a Seminar on Natural Fertility*, edited by Henri Leridon and Jane A. Menken. Ordina Editions, Liège, Belgium (for the International Union for the Scientific Study of Population), pp. 149–194.

Janossy, George, J. Alero Thomas, Fred J. Bollum, Sylvia Granger, Giovanni Pizzolo, Kenneth F. Bradstock, Leslie Wong, Andrew McMichael, K. Ganeshaguru, and A. V. Hoffbrand (1980). The human thymic microenvironment: An immunohistologic study. *Journal of Immunology* **125**, 202–212.

Janowitz, Barbara, JoAnn Henderson Lewis, Allan M. Parnell, Fouad W. Hefnawi, M. N. Younis, and Gamal Abou Serour (1981). Breast-feeding and child survival in Egypt. *Journal of Biosocial Science* **13**, 287–297.

Jason, Janine M., Phillip Nieburg, and James S. Marks (1984). Mortality and infectious disease associated with infant-feeding practices in developing countries. *Pediatrics* **74**, 702–727.

Jathar, V. S., S. A. Kamath, M. N. Parikh, D. V. Rege, and R. S. Satoskar (1970). Maternal milk and serum vitamin B_{12}, folic acid, and protein levels in Indian subjects. *Archives of Diseases in Childhood* **45**, 236–241.

Jayme-Ho, Teresa (1976). Time allocation, home production and labor force participation of married women: An exploratory survey. Institute of Economic Development and Research Discussion Paper no. 76-8. University of the Philippines, [Dillman, Quezon City].

Jelliffe, Derrick Brian (1966). *The Assessment of the Nutritional Status of the Community* (with Special Reference to Field Surveys in Developing Regions of the World). World Health Organization Monograph Series no. 53. Geneva.

Jelliffe, Derrick Brian, and E. F. Patrice Jelliffe (1971). The uniqueness of human milk. An overview. *American Journal of Clinical Nutrition* **24**, 1013–1024.

Jelliffe, Derrick Brian, and E. F. Patrice Jelliffe (1978a). *Human Milk in the Modern World: Psychosocial, Nutritional, and Economic Significance*. Oxford University Press, Oxford, England.

Jelliffe, Derrick Brian, and E. F. Patrice Jelliffe (1978b). The volume and composition of human milk in poorly nourished communities. A review. *American Journal of Clinical Nutrition* **31**, 492–515.

Jelliffe, E. F. Patrice (1976). Maternal nutrition and lactation. In *Breast Feeding and the Mother*. Ciba Foundation Symposium 45 (n.s.). Elsevier/Excerpta Medica/North Holland, Amsterdam, pp. 119–143.

Jenness, Robert (1974). The composition of milk. In *Lactation. A Comprehensive Treatise*. Vol. 3, *Nutrition and Biochemistry of Milk/Maintenance*, edited by Bruce L. Larson and Vearl R. Smith. Academic Press, New York, pp. 3–107.

Jenness, Robert (1979). The composition of human milk. *Seminars in Perinatology* **3**, 225–239.

Jensen, Robert G., Mary M. Hagerty, and Kathleen E. McMahon (1978). Lipids of human milk and infant formulas: A review. *American Journal of Clinical Nutrition* **31**, 990–1016.

Jimenez, Marcia Houdek, and Niles A. Newton (1979). Activity and work during pregnancy and the postpartum period: A cross cultural study of 202 societies. *American Journal of Obstetrics and Gynecology* **135**, 171–176.

Johnson, Dianne F., Gene L. France, Daniel J. Marmer, and Russell W. Steele (1980). Bactericidal mechanisms of human breast milk leukocytes. *Infection and Immunity* **28**, 314–318.

Johnston, Francis E., Alex F. Roche, Lawrence M. Schell, and Norman B. Wettenhall (1975). Critical weight at menarche. *American Journal of Diseases of Children* **129**, 19–23.

Johnston, Judith (1977). The household context of infant feeding practices in south Trinidad. *Lactation Review* **2**, 412–423.

Jollès, Pierre, and Jacqueline Jollès (1961). Lysozyme from human milk. *Nature* **192**, 1187–1188.

Josephs, Shelby H., and Rebecca H. Buckley (1980). Serum IgD concentrations in normal infants, children, and adults and in patients with elevated IgE. *Journal of Pediatrics* **96**, 417–420.

Kanaaneh, Hatim (1972). The relationship of bottle feeding to malnutrition and gastroenteritis in a pre-industrial setting. *Journal of Tropical Pediatrics and Environmental Child Health* **18**, 302–306.

Kanawati, Abdallah A., and Donald S. McLaren (1973). Failure to thrive in Lebanon. II. An investigation of the causes. *Acta Paediatrica Scandinavica* **62**, 571–576.

Karmarkar, M. G., J. Kapur, A. D. Deodhar, and C. V. Ramakrishnan (1959). Diet survey of lactating women in different socio-economic groups and the effects of socio-economic status and stage of lactation on the proximate principles and essential amino acids of human milk. *Indian Journal of Medical Research* **47**, 344–351.

Katona-Apte, Judit (1977). The socio-cultural aspects of food avoidance in a low-income population in Tamiland, South India. *Journal of Tropical Pediatrics and Environmental Child Health* **23**, 83–90.

Kaur, Paramjeet, G. Srivastava, and Kunal Saha (1979). Immunological response of low birth weight babies from birth to 6 months. *Indian Pediatrics* **16**, 985–996.

Kenny, Jean F., Mary I. Boesman, and Richard H. Michaels (1967). Bacterial and viral coproantibodies in breast-fed infants. *Pediatrics* **39**, 202–213.

Khan, M. U. (1984). Breastfeeding, growth and diarrhoea in rural Bangladesh children. *Human Nutrition: Clinical Nutrition* **38C**, 113–119.

Khin-Maung-Naing, Tin-Tin-Oo, Kywe-Thein, and Nwe-New-Hlaing (1980). Study on lactation performance of Burmese mothers. *American Journal of Clinical Nutrition* **33**, 2665–2668.

Kingston, Michael E. (1975). Biochemical disturbances in breast-fed infants with gastroenteritis and dehydration. *Journal of Pediatrics* **82**, 1073–1081.

Kinoshita, Kenichiro, Shigeo Hino, Tatsuhiko Amagasaki, Shuichi Ikeda, Yasuaki Yamada, Junji Suzuyama, Saburo Momita, Kazuhiro Toriya, Shimeru Kamihira, and Michito Ichimaru (1984). Demonstrations of adult T-cell leukemia virus antigen in milk from three sero-positive mothers. *Gann* **75**, 103–105.

Klein, Robert B., Thomas J. Fischer, Sherrie E. Gard, Michael Biberstein, Kenneth C. Rich, and Richard E. Stiehm (1977). Decreased mononuclear and polymorphonuclear chemotaxis in human newborns, infants, and young children. *Pediatrics* **60**, 467–472.

Kleinbaum, David G., Lawrence L. Kupper, and Hal Morgenstern (1982). *Epidemiologic Research: Principles and Quantitative Methods*. Lifetime Learning Publications, Belmont, Calif.

Knodel, John (1977). Breast-feeding and population growth. *Science* **198**(16 Dec.), 1111–1115

Koldovsky, Otakar (1980). Minireview: Hormones in milk. *Life Sciences* **26**, 1833–1836.

Kovar, Mary Grace, Mary K. Serdula, James S. Marks, and David W. Fraser (1984). Review of the epidemiological evidence for an association between infant feeding and infant health. *Pediatrics* **74**, 615–638.

Krámer, M., K. Szöke, K. Lindner, and R. Tarján (1965). The effect of different factors on the composition of human milk and its variations. III. Effect of dietary fats on the lipid composition of human milk. *Nutritio et Dieta* **7**, 71–79.

Krugman, Saul (1975). Vertical transmission of Hepatitis B and breast-feeding. *The Lancet* **2**(8 Nov.), 916.

Kusin, Jane A., Sri Kardjati, C. De With, and I. K. Sudibia (1979). Nutrition and nutritional status of rural women in East Java. *Tropical and Geographical Medicine* **31**, 571–585.

Lakdawala, Dilnawaz R., and Elsie M. Widdowson (1977). Vitamin-D in human milk. *The Lancet* **1**(22 Jan.), 167–168.

Last, John M., ed. (1983). *A Dictionary of Epidemiology*. Oxford University Press, New York.

Laukaran, Virginia Hight (1981). Contraceptive choices for lactating women: Suggestions for postpartum family planning. In "Breast-feeding program, policy and research issues," edited by Edward C. Baer and Beverly Winikoff. *Studies in Family Planning* **12**, 156–163.

Lawton, Alexander R., and Max D. Cooper (1979). B cell ontogeny—immunoglobulin genes and their expression. *Pediatrics* **64**(suppl.), 750–757.

Lee, Elisa T. (1980). *Statistical Methods for Survival Data Analysis*. Lifetime Learning Publications, Belmont, Calif.

Lee, Jenny Green, and Giorgio Solimano (1981). Including mothers in the design of infant feeding research. *Studies in Family Planning* **12**, 173–176.

Lengemann, F. W. (1959). The site of action of lactose in the enhancement of calcium utilization. *Journal of Nutrition* **69**, 23–27.

Lepage, Phillipe, Christophe Munyakazi, and Phillipe Hennart (1981). Breastfeeding and hospital mortality in children in Rwanda. *The Lancet* **2** (22 Aug.), 409–411.

Leridon, Henri (1977). *Human Fertility: The Basic Components*, translated by Judith F. Helzner. University of Chicago Press, Chicago.

Lewis-Jones, D. I., and G. J. Reynolds (1983). A suggested role for precolostrum in preterm and sick newborn infants. *Acta Paediatrica Scandinavica* **72**, 13–17.

Liebhaber, Myron, Norman J. Lewiston, Maria Teresa Asquith, Lynne Olds-Arroyo, and Philip Sunshine (1977). Alterations of lymphocytes and of antibody content of human milk after processing. *Journal of Pediatrics* **91**, 897–900.

Lindblad, B. S., and Razia J. Rahimtoola (1974). A pilot study of the quality of human milk in a lower socio-economic group in Karachi, Pakistan. *Acta Paediatrica Scandinavica* **63**, 125–128.

Liskin, Laurie S. (1981). Periodic abstinence: How well do new approaches work? *Population Reports*, ser. I, no. 3.

London, D. R., M. R. Glass, R. W. Shaw, W. R. Butt, and R. Logan-Edwards (1977). The modulation by ovarian hormones of gonadotrophin release in hyperprolactinaemic women. In *Prolactin and Human Reproduction, Proceedings of the Serono Symposia*. Vol. 11, edited by Pier Giorgio Crosignani and Claude Robyn. Academic Press, London, pp. 119–124.

Lubens, R., M. Soderberg-Warner, S. Gard, and E. Richard Stiehm (1980). Diminished T cell cytotoxicity in newborns and young children. *Clinical Research* **28**, 109A.

Lucas, Alan, Penny J. Lucas, and J. David Baum (1980). The nipple-shield sampling system: A device for measuring the dietary intake of breast-fed infants. *Early Human Development* **4**, 365–372.

Lunn, Peter G., Andrew M. Prentice, Steven Austin, and Roger G. Whitehead (1980). Influence of maternal diet on plasma-prolactin levels during lactation. *The Lancet* **1**(22 Mar.), 623–625.

Lunn, Peter G., Michael Watkinson, Andrew M. Prentice, Peter Morrell, Steven Austin, and Roger G. Whitehead (1981). Maternal nutrition and lactational amenorrhea. *The Lancet* **1**(27 June), 1428–1429.

McCance, R. A., and Widdowson, Elsie M. (1962). Nutrition and Growth. *Proceedings of the Royal Society of London*. Series B. *Biological Sciences* **156**, 326–337.

McCann, Margaret F., Laurie S. Liskin, Phyllis T. Piotrow, Ward Rinehart, and Gordon Fox (1981). Breast-feeding, fertility and family planning. *Population Reports*, ser. J, no. 24.

McClelland, D. B. L., R. R. Samson, D. M. Parkin, and D. J. C. Shearman (1972). Bacterial agglutination studies with secretory IgA prepared from human gastrointestinal secretions and colostrum. *Gut* **13**, 450–458.

McGuire, Judith Snavely (1979). Seasonal changes in woman's energy expenditure and work patterns of rural Guatemalan peasants. Ph.D. dissertation, Massachusetts Institute of Technology, Cambridge.

McKenzie, Herman I., Howard G. Lovell, Kenneth L. Standard, and William E. Miall (1967). Child mortality in Jamaica. *Milbank Memorial Fund Quarterly* **45**, 303–320.

McKigney, John I. (1968). Economic aspects of infant feeding practices in the West Indies. *Journal of Tropical Pediatrics* **14**, 55–59.

McKigney, John I. (1971). The uniqueness of human milk: Economic aspects. *American Journal of Clinical Nutrition* **24**, 1005–1012.

McMillan, Julia A., Stephen A. Landaw, and Frank A. Oski (1976). Iron sufficiency in breast-fed infants and the availability of iron from human milk. *Pediatrics* **58**, 686–691.

McMurray, David N., Scott A. Loomis, Lawrence J. Casazza, Humberto Rey, and Reynaldo Miranda (1981). Development of impaired cell-mediated immunity in mild and moderate malnutrition. *American Journal of Clinical Nutrition* **34**, 68–77.

McNatty, K. P., R. S. Sawers, and Alan S. McNeilly (1974). A possible role for prolactin in control of steroid secretion by the human Graafian follicle. *Nature* **250**, 653–655.

McNeilly, Alan S. (1977). Physiology of lactation. *Journal of Biosocial Science* (suppl. 4), 5–21.

McNeilly, Alan S., Peter W. Howie, and Mary J. Houston (1980). Relationship of feeding patterns, prolactin, and resumption of ovulation postpartum. In *Research Frontiers in Fertility Regulation: Proceedings of an International Workshop on Research Frontiers in Fertility Regulation, Mexico City, Mexico, February 11–14, 1980*, edited by Gerald I. Zatuchni, Miriam H. Labbok, and John J. Sciarra. Harper and Row, Hagerstown, Md., pp. 102–116.

McNeilly, Alan S., P. G. Lunn, and Hernán Delgado (1981). The role of prolactin on the contraceptive effect of lactation, and the influence of breast-feeding practices of maternal dietary status. In *Maternal Diet, Breast-feeding Capacity, and Lactational Infertility*, edited by Roger G. Whitehead. Report of a joint UNU/WHO workshop held in Cambridge, United Kingdom, 9–11 March 1981. The United Nations University, Tokyo, pp. 72–80.

McNeilly, Alan S., A. F. Glasier, Peter W. Howie, Mary J. Houston, A. Cook, and H. Boyle (1983). Fertility after childbirth: Pregnancy associated with breast feeding. *Clinical Endocrinology* **19**, 167–173.

Malkani, Parvati K., and Janki J. Mirchandani (1960). Menstruation during lactation. A clinical study. *Journal of Obstetrics and Gynaecology of India* **11**, 9–22.

Mamunes, Peter, Paul E. Prince, Nancy H. Thornton, Patricia A. Hunt, and Elizabeth S. Hitchcock (1976). Intellectual deficits after transient tyrosinemia in the term neonate. *Pediatrics* **57**, 675–680.

Manerikar, Shanta S., A. N. Malaviya, Mehar Ban Singh, Premawathi Rajgopalan, and R. Kumar (1976). Immune status and BCG vaccination in newborns with intra-uterine growth retardation. *Clinical and Experimental Immunology* **26**, 173–175.

Mannheimer, Edgar (1955). Mortality of breast fed and bottle fed infants: A comparative study. *Acta Geneticae et Statistica Medicae* **5**, 134–163.

Martinez, Gilbert A., and John P. Nalezienski (1981). 1980 update: The recent trend in breast-feeding. *Pediatrics* **67**, 260–263.

Martorell, Reynaldo, and Chloe O'Gara (1984). Breastfeeding, infant health and socioeconomic status. Paper presented at the symposium, Biocultural Factors Affecting Infant Feeding and Growth, annual meeting of the American Anthropological Association, 18 November, Denver.

Martorell, Reynaldo, and Charles Yarbrough (1983). The energy cost of diarrheal diseases and other common illnesses in children. In *Diarrhea and Nutrition. Intractions, Mechanisms, and Interventions*, edited by Lincoln C. Chen and Nevin S. Scrimshaw. Plenum, New York, pp. 125–154.

Mata, Leonardo J., and Richard G. Wyatt (1971). The uniqueness of human milk. Host resistance to infection. *American Journal of Clinical Nutrition* **24**, 976–986.

Mata, Leonardo J., Franklin Jiménez, Miriam Cordón, Roberto Rosales, Erick Prera, Roberto E. Schneider, and Fernando Veteri (1972). Gastrointestinal flora of children with protein-calorie malnutrition. *American Journal of Clinical Nutrition* **25**, 1118–1126.

Mata, Leonardo J., Richard A. Kromal, Juan J. Urrutia, and Bertha Garcia (1977). Effect of infection on food intake and the nutritional state: Perspectives as viewed from the village. *American Journal of Clinical Nutrition* **30**, 1215–1227.

Mata, Leonardo J., Juan J. Urrutia, and John E. Gordon (1967). Diarrhoeal disease in a cohort of Guatemalan village children observed from birth to age two years. *Tropical and Geographical Medicine* **19**, 247–257.

Mayes, Harry W. (1947). Epidemic diarrhea in the newborn. The relation between breast and bottle feeding and the early development of the proper intestinal flora. *American Journal of Obstetrics and Gynecology* **53**, 285–289.

Maynard, James E., and Laurel M. Hammes (1970). A study of growth, morbidity and mortality among Eskimo infants of western Alaska. *Bulletin of the World Health Organization* **42**, 613–622.

Mead Johnson Laboratories (1977). *Infant Formulas: Handbook*. [Mead Johnson & Co., Evansville, Ind.]

Menken, Jane A., James Trussell, and Susan Watkins (1981). The nutrition-fertility link: An evaluation of the evidence. *Journal of Interdisciplinary History* **11**, 425–441.

Michael, J. Gabriel, Raymond Ringenback, and Susan Hottenstein (1971). The antimicrobial activity of human colostral antibody in the newborn. *Journal of Infectious Diseases* **124**, 445–448.

Michaels, Richard H. (1965). Studies of antiviral factors in human milk and serum. *Journal of Immunology* **94**, 262–271.

Miller, Michael E. (1971). Chemotactic function in the human neonate: Humoral and cellular aspects. *Pediatric Research* **5**, 487–492.

Miller, Michael E. (1978). *Host Defenses in the Human Neonate. Monographs on Neonatology.* Grune & Stratton, New York.

Miller, Michael E., and E. Richard Stiehm (1983). Immunology and resistance to infection. In *Infectious Diseases of the Fetus and Newborn Infant*, edited by Jack S. Remington and Jerome O. Klein. 2d ed. Saunders, Philadelphia, pp. 27–68.

Millman, Sara (1984). Breastfeeding and infant mortality—Untangling the complex web of causality. Population Studies and Training Center Working Paper no. WP-84-03. Brown University, Providence, R.I.

Millman, Sara (1985). Breastfeeding and contraception: Why the inverse association? *Studies in Family Planning* **16**, 61–75.

Miranda, Reynaldo, Nancy G. Saravia, Ruben Ackerman, Neva Murphy, Stephen Berman, and David N. McMurray (1983). Effect of maternal nutritional status on immunological substances in human colostrum and milk. *American Journal of Clinical Nutrition* **37**, 632–640.

Mittal, S. K., A. Kanwar, A. Varghese, and V. G. Ramachandran (1983). Gut flora in breast and bottle fed infants with and without diarrhea. *Indian Pediatrics* **20**, 21–26.

Mohr, John A., Richard Leu, and Wynn Mabry (1970). Colostral leukocytes. *Journal of Surgical Oncology* **2**, 163–167.

Molla, A. Majid, Ayesha Molla, S. A. Sarker, and M. Mujiber Rahaman (1983). Food intake during and after recovery from diarrhea in children. In *Diarrhea and Malnutrition: Interactions, Mechanisms, and Interventions*, edited by Lincoln C. Chen and Nevin

S. Scrimshaw. Sponsored by the United Nations University, Tokyo, Japan. New York, Plenum, pp. 113–123.

Moro, Itaru, Sylvia S. Crago, and Jiri Mestecky (1983). Localization of IgA and IgM in human colostral elements using immunoelectron microscopy. *Journal of Clinical Immunology* **3**, 382–391.

Mosley, W. Henry (1979). The effects of nutrition on natural fertility. In *Natural Fertility: Patterns and Determinants of Natural Fertility: Proceedings of a Seminar on Natural Fertility*, edited by Henri Leridon and Jane A. Menken. Ordina Editions, Liège, Belgium (for the International Union for the Scientific Study of Population), pp. 83–105.

Mouton, R. P., J. W. Stoop, R. E. Ballieux, and N. A. J. Mul (1970). Pneumococcal antibodies in IgA of serum and external secretions. *Clinical and Experimental in Immunology* **7**, 201–210.

Murillo, G. J., and Armond S. Goldman (1970). The cells of human colostrum. II. Synthesis of IgA and β1c. *Pediatric Research* **4**, 71–75.

Murphy, J. F., M. L. Neale, and N. Matthews (1983). Antimicrobial properties of preterm breast milk cells. *Archives of Disease in Childhood* **58**, 198–200.

Myers, Martin G., Samuel J. Fomon, Franklin P. Koontz, Gail A. McGuiness, Peter A. Lachenbruch, and Rachel Hollingshead (1984). Respiratory and gastrointestinal illnesses in breast- and formula-fed infants. *American Journal of Disease of Children* **138**, 629–632.

Naish, F. Charlotte (1951). Successful breast-feeding. *British Medical Journal* **1**(24 Mar.), 607–610.

Naismith, D. J., Susan P. Deeprose, G. Supramaniam, and M. J. H. Williams (1978). Reappraisal of linoleic acid requirement of the young infant, with particular regard to use of modified cows' milk formulae. *Archives of Disease in Childhood* **53**, 845–849.

National Center for Health Statistics (1976). NCHS growth charts, 1976. *Monthly Vital Statistics Report* **25**, no. 3 suppl.

National Research Council. Assembly of Life Sciences. Division of Biological Sciences. Food and Nutrition Board. Committee on Dietary Allowances (1980). *Recommended Dietary Allowances*. 9th rev. ed. National Academy of Sciences, Washington, D.C.

National Research Council. Committee on Maternal Nutrition (1970). *Maternal Nutrition and the Course of Pregnancy*. National Academy of Sciences, Washington, D.C.

Nayman, Rhona, Mary Ellen Thomson, Charles R. Sriver, and Carol L. Clow (1979). Observations on the composition of milk-substitute products for the treatment of inborn errors of amino acid metabolism. Comparisons with human milk. A proposal to rationalize nutrient content of treatment products. *American Journal of Clinical Nutrition* **32**, 1279–1289.

NCHS. See National Center for Health Statistics.

Nelson, Robert D., and Richard W. Leu (1975). Macrophage requirement for production of guinea pig migration inhibitory factor (MIF) in vitro. *Journal of Immunology* **114**, 606–609.

Neumann, Charlotte G. (1979). Reference data. In *Human Nutrition. A Comprehensive Treatise*. Vol 2. *Nutrition and Growth*, edited by Derrick Brian Jelliffe and E. F. Patrice Jelliffe. Plenum, New York, pp. 299–327.

Newton, Michael A., and Niles A. Newton (1962). The normal course and management of lactation. *Clinical Obstetrics and Gynecology* **5**(1), 44–63.

Newton, Niles A. (1973). Interrelationships between sexual responsiveness, birth, and breast feeding. In *Contemporary Sexual Behavior: Critical Issues in the 1970's*, edited by Joseph Zubin and John Money. Johns Hopkins University Press, Baltimore, pp. 77–98.

NFP. See Nutrition Foundation of the Philippines.

Nichols, Buford L., and Veda N. Nichols (1979). Lactation. *Advances in Pediatrics* **26**, 137–161.

Noel, Gordon L., Han K. Suh, and Andrew G. Frantz (1974). Prolactin release during nursing and breast stimulation in postpartum and nonpostpartum subjects. *Journal of Clinical Endocrinology and Metabolism* **38**, 413–423.

Noel, Gordon L., Han K. Suh, J. Gilbert Stone, and Andrew G. Frantz (1972). Human prolactin and growth hormone release during surgery and other conditions of stress. *Journal of Clinical Endocrinology and Metabolism* **35**, 840–851.

Nordbring, Folke (1957). The appearance of antistreptolysin and antistaphylolysin in human colostrum. *Acta Paediatrica* **46**, 481–496.

Norgan, N. G., A. Ferro-Luzzi, and John Valentine George Andrew Durnin (1974). The energy and nutrient intake and the energy expenditure of 204 New Guinean adults. *Philosophical Transactions of the Royal Society of London* **B268**, 309–348.

Notzon, Francis (1984). Trends in infant feeding in developed countries. *Pediatrics* **74**, 648–666.

NRC. See National Research Council.

Nutrition Foundation of the Philippines, Field Service Section (1977). Dietary survey among pregnant and lactating women in a resettlement. 2. Twenty-four-hour recall. *Philippine Journal of Nutrition* **30**, 119–122.

Nyhan, William L., and Morris A. Wessel (1954). Neonatal growth in weight of normal infants on four different feeding regimens. *Pediatrics* **14**, 442–447.

Oakley, J. R. (1977). Differences in subcutaneous fat in breast- and formula-fed infants. *Archives of Diseases in Childhood* **52**, 79–80.

O'Connor, P. A. (1978). Failure to thrive with breast-feeding. *Clinical Pediatrics* **17**, 833–835.

O'Gara, Chloe, and Carl Kendall (in press). Fluids and powders: Options for infant feeding.

Ogra, S. S., and Pearay L. Ogra (1978). Immunologic aspects of human colostrum and milk. II. Characteristics of lymphocyte reactivity and distribution of E-rosette forming cells at different times after the onset of lactation. *Journal of Pediatrics* **92**, 550–555.

Ogra, S. S., D. Weintraub, and Pearay L. Ogra (1977). Immunologic aspects of human colostrum and milk. III. Fate and absorption of cellular and soluble components in the gastrointestinal tract of the newborn. *Journal of Immunology* **119**, 245–248.

Omran, Abdel Rahim, and C. C. Standley (1976). *Family Formation Patterns and Health: An International Collaborative Study in India, Iran, Lebanon, Philippines, and Turkey.* World Health Organization, Geneva.

Osborn, John J., Joseph Dancis, and Juan F. Julia (1952). Studies of the immunology of the newborn infant. 1. Age and antibody production. *Pediatrics* **9**, 736–744.

Oski, Frank A., and Stephen A. Landaw (1980). Inhibition of iron absorption from human milk by baby food. *American Journal of Diseases of Children* **134**, 459–460.

Osteria, Trinidad S. (1973). Lactation and postpartum amenorrhea in a rural community. *Acta Medica Philippina* **9**(4), 144–151.

Osteria, Trinidad S. (1978). Variations in fertility with breast-feeding practice and contraception in urban Filipino women: Implications for a nutrition program. In *Nutrition and Human Reproduction*, edited by W. Henry Mosley. Plenum Press, New York, pp. 411–432.

Osteria, Trinidad S. (1983). Lactation and childhood mortality in an urban area in the Philippines. *Philippine Journal of Nutrition* **36**, 95–103.

Otnaess, Anne-Brit, and Ivar Ørstavik (1980). The effect of human milk fractions on rotavirus in relation to the secretory IgA content. *Acta Pathologica et Microbiologica Scandinavica* **88C**, 15–21.

Owen, George M., Philip J. Garry, Elizabeth M. Hooper, Barbara A. Gilbert, and Dorothy Pathak (1981). Iron nutriture of infants exclusively breast-fed the first five months. *Journal of Pediatrics* **99**, 237–240.

Packard, Vernal S. (1982). *Human Milk and Infant Formula.* Food Science and Technology

Monographs Series, edited by George F. Stewart, Bernard S. Schweigert, and John Hawthorn. Academic Press, New York.

Park, B. H., B. Holmes, and R. A. Good (1970). Metabolic activities in leukocytes of newborn infants. *Journal of Pediatrics* **76**, 237–241.

Parmely, Michael J., Alan E. Beer, and Rupert E. Billingham (1976). In vitro studies on the T-lymphocyte population of human milk. *Journal of Experimental Medicine* **144**, 358–370.

Pasricha, Swaran (1958). A survey of dietary intake in a group of poor, pregnant and lactating women. *Indian Journal of Medical Research* **46**, 605–609.

Passmore, Reginald, B. M. Nichol, and M. Narayana Rao in collaboration with George H. Beaton and E. M. DeMayer (1974). *Handbook on Human Nutritional Requirements.* FAO Nutritional Series, no. 28. WHO Monograph Series, no. 61. Food and Agriculture Organization of the United Nations and World Health Organization, Rome.

Paul, Alison A., and Elizabeth M. Müller (1980). Seasonal variations in dietary intakes in pregnant and lactating women in a rural Gambian village. In *Maternal Nutrition during Pregnancy and Lactation: A Nestlé Foundation Workshop.* Lutry/Lausanne, April 26th and 27th 1969, edited by Hugo Aebi and Roger G. Whitehead. Nestlé Foundation Publication Series no. 1. Hans Huber, Bern, pp. 105–116.

Paul, Alison A., Elisabeth M. Müller, and Roger G. Whitehead (1979a). The quantitative effects of maternal dietary energy intake on pregnancy and lactation in rural Gambian women. *Transactions of the Royal Society of Tropical Medicine and Hygiene* **73**, 686–692.

Paul, Alison, Elisabeth M. Müller, and Roger G. Whitehead (1979b). Seasonal variations in energy intake, body-weight and skinfold thickness in pregnant and lactating women in rural Gambia. *Proceedings of the Nutrition Society* **38**, 28A.

Pekkarinen, Maija (1970). Methodology in the collection of food consumption data. *World Review of Nutrition and Dietetics* **12**, 145–171.

Pérez, Alfredo (1979). Lactational amenorrhea and natural family planning. In *Human Ovulation: Mechanisms, Prediction, Detection and Induction*, edited by E. S. E. Hafez. Human Reproductive Medicine, vol. 3. North-Holland, Amsterdam, pp. 501–513.

Pérez, Alfredo, Patricio Velo, George S. Masnick, and Robert G. Potter (1972). First ovulation after childbirth: The effect of breast-feeding. *American Journal of Obstetrics and Gynecology* **114**, 1041–1047.

Petros-Barvazian, Angèle, and Moishe Béhar (1979). Low birth-weight—A major global problem. In *Birth-weight Distribution—An Indicator of Social Development*, edited by Göran Sterky and Lotta Mellander. SAREC Report no. R:2 1978. Swedish Agency for Research Cooperation with Developing Countries, Stockholm, pp. 9–15.

Picciano, Mary Frances, and Ronald H. Deering (1980). The influence of feeding regimens on iron status during infancy. *American Journal of Clinical Nutrition* **33**, 746–753.

Picciano, Mary Frances, Helen Andrews Guthrie, and Dennis M. Sheehe (1978). The cholesterol content of human milk. A variable constituent among women and within the same woman. *Clinical Pediatrics* **17**, 359–362.

Pickering, Larry K., Thomas G. Cleary, and Richard M. Caprioli (1983). Inhibition of human polymorphonuclear leukocyte function by components of human colostrum and mature milk. *Infection and Immunity* **40**, 8–15.

Piletz, J. E., and Roger E. Ganschow (1979). Is acrodermatitis enteropathica related to the absence of zinc binding ligand in bovine milk? *American Journal of Clinical Nutrition* **32**, 275–277.

Pitt, Jane (1979). The milk mononuclear phagocyte. *Pediatrics* **64**(suppl.), 745–749.

Pitt, Jane, Barbara Barlow, and William C. Heird (1977). Protection against experimental necrotizing enterocolitis by maternal milk. I. Role of milk leukocytes. *Pediatric Research* **11**, 906–909.

Pittard, William B., III (1979). Breast milk immunology. A frontier in infant nutrition. *American Journal of Diseases of Children* **133**, 83–87.

Pittard, William B., III, S. H. Polmar, and A. A. Fanaroff (1977). The breastmilk macrophage: A potential vehicle for immunoglobulin transport. *RES: Journal of Reticuloendothelial Society* **22**, 597–603.

Plank, S. J., and M. L. Milanesi (1973). Infant feeding and infant mortality in rural Chile. *Bulletin of the World Health Organization* **48**, 203–210.

Poland, Ronald L., and Sanford N. Cohen (1980). The contamination of the food chain in Michigan with PBB: The breast-feeding question. In *Drug and Chemical Risks to the Fetus and Newborn: Proceedings of a Symposium Held in New York May 21 and 22, 1979*, edited by Richard A. Schwartz and Sumner J. Yaffe. Progress in Clinical and Biological Research vol. 36. Liss, New York, pp. 129–137.

Popkin, Barry M. (1978). Economic determinants of breast-feeding behavior: The case of rural households in Laguna, Philippines. In *Nutrition and Human Reproduction*, edited by W. Henry Mosley. Plenum, New York, pp. 461–497.

Popkin, Barry M., and Michael C. Latham (1973). The limitations and dangers of commerciogenic nutritious foods. *American Journal of Clinical Nutrition* **26**, 1015–1023.

Popkin, Barry M., Richard E. Bilsborrow, and John S. Akin (1982). Breast-feeding patterns in low-income countries. *Science* **218**(10 Dec.), 1088–1093.

Poplack, David G., and R. Michael Blaese (1980). The mononuclear phagocytic system. In *Immunologic Disorders in Infants and Children*, edited by E. Richard Stiehm and Vincent A. Fulginiti. Saunders, Philadelphia, pp. 109–126.

Potter, Julia M., and Paul J. Nestel (1976). The effects of dietary fatty acids and cholesterol on the milk lipids of lactating women and the plasma cholesterol of breast-fed infants. *American Journal of Clinical Nutrition* **29**, 54–60.

Potter, Robert G., Jr., and Frances E. Kobrin (1981). Distributions of amenorrhea and anovulation. *Population Studies* **35**, 85–99.

Potter, Robert G., Jr., Frances E. Kobrin, and Raymond L. Langsten (1979). Evaluating acceptance strategies for timing of postpartum contraception. *Studies in Family Planning* **10**, 151–160.

Prader, A., James M. Tanner, and G. A. von Harnack (1963). Catch-up growth following illness or starvation: An example of developmental canalization in man. *Journal of Pediatrics* **62**, 646–659.

Prema, Krishnamurthy, and M. Ravindranath (1982). The effect of breastfeeding supplements on the return of fertility. *Studies in Family Planning* **13**, 293–296.

Prema, Krishnamurthy, A. Nadamuni Naidu, and S. Neela Kumari (1979). Lactation and fertility. *American Journal of Clinical Nutrition* **32**, 1298–1303.

Prema, Krishnamurthy, R. Madhavapeddi, B. A. Ramalakshmi, S. Samyukta, and S. Babu (1981). Effect of lactation on maternal haemoglobin levels. *Nutrition Reports International* **24**, 825–830.

Prema, Krishnamurthy, A. Nadamuni Naidu, S. Neela Kumari, and B. A. Ramalakshmi (1980). Nutrition-fertility interaction in lactating women of low income groups. *British Journal of Nutrition* **45**, 461–467.

Prentice, Andrew M. (1980). Variations in maternal dietary intake, birthweight and breast-milk output in the Gambia. In *Maternal Nutrition during Pregnancy and Lactation: A Nestlé Foundation Workshop: Lutry/Lausanne, April 26th and 27th 1979*, edited by Hugo Aebi and Roger G. Whitehead. Nestlé Foundation Publication Series no. 1. Hans Huber, Bern, pp. 167–183.

Prentice, Ann, Andrew M. Prentice, T. J. Cole, and Roger G. Whitehead (1983a). Determinants of variations in breast milk protective factor concentrations of rural Gambian mothers. *Archives of Disease in Childhood* **58**, 518–522.

Prentice, Andrew M., Ann Prentice, W. H. Lamb, Peter G. Lunn, and Steven Austin (1983b).

Metabolic consequences of fasting during Ramadan in pregnant and lactating women. *Human Nutrition: Clinical Nutrition* **37C**, 283–294.

Prentice, Andrew M., Roger G. Whitehead, Susan B. Roberts, and Alison A. Paul (1981). Long-term energy balance in child-bearing Gambian women. *American Journal of Clinical Nutrition* **34**, 2790–2799.

Prentice, Andrew M., Roger G. Whitehead, Susan B. Roberts, Alison A. Paul, Michael Watkinson, Ann Prentice, and Anne A. Watkinson (1980). Dietary supplementation of Gambian nursing mothers and lactational performance. *The Lancet* **2**(25 Oct.), 886–888.

Pullan, C. R., G. L. Toms, A. J. Martin, P. S. Gardner, J. K. G. Webb, and D. R. Appleton (1980). Breast-feeding and respiratory syncytial virus infection. *British Medical Journal* **281**(18 Oct.), 1034–1036.

Rajalakshmi, R. (1971). Reproductive performance of poor Indian women on a low plane of nutrition. *Tropical and Geographical Medicine* **23**, 117–125.

Rajalakshmi, R. (1980). Gestation and lactation performance in relation to the plane of maternal nutrition. In *Maternal Nutrition during Pregnancy and Lactation: A Nestlé Foundation Workshop: Lutry/Lausanne, April 26th and 27th 1979*, edited by Hugo Aebi and Roger G. Whitehead. Nestlé Foundation Publication Series no. 1. Hans Huber, Bern, pp. 184–202.

Rassin, David K., John A. Sturman, and Gerald E. Gaull (1978). Taurine and other free amino acids in milk of man and other animals. *Early Human Development* **2**, 1–13.

Read, W. W. C., Phyllis G. Lutz, and Anahid Tashjian (1965). Human milk lipids. II. The influence of dietary carbohydrates and fat on the fatty acids of mature milk. A study in four ethnic groups. *American Journal of Clinical Nutrition* **17**, 180–183.

Reddy, Vinodini C., C. Bhaskaram, N. Raghuramulu, and V. Jagadeesan (1977). Antimicrobial factors in human milk. *Acta Paediatrica Scandinavica* **66**, 229–232.

Reeve, Lorraine E., Russell W. Chesney, and Hector F. DeLuca (1982). Vitamin D of human milk: Identification of biologically active forms. *American Journal of Clinical Nutrition* **36**, 122–126.

Reeves, Jaxk. (1979). Estimating fatness. *Science* **204**(25 May), 881.

Reiser, Raymond, and Zvi Sidelman (1972). Control of serum cholesterol homeostasis by cholesterol in the milk of the suckling rat. *Journal of Nutrition* **102**, 1009–1016.

Roberts, D. W. (1980). Growth of breast fed and bottle fed infants. *New Zealand Medical Journal* **92**, 45–46.

Roberts, S. A., and D. L. J. Freed (1977). Neonatal IgA secretion enhanced by breastfeeding. *The Lancet* **2**(26 Nov.), 1131.

Roberts, S. A., G. Wincup, and D. A. Harries (1980). Mucosal receptor for IgA in the breast-fed neonate. *Early Human Development* **4**, 161–166.

Robinson, Margaret (1951). Infant morbidity and mortality. A study of 3266 infants. *The Lancet* **1**, 788–794.

Roddey, O. F., Edward S. Martin, and Raymond L. Swetenburg (1981). Critical weight loss and malnutrition in breast-fed infants: Four case reports. *American Journal of Diseases of Children* **135**, 597–599.

Rogan, Walter J., Anna Bagniewska, and Terri Damstra (1980). Pollutants in breast milk. *New England Journal of Medicine* **302**(26 June), 1450–1453.

Rosa, Franz W. (1975). The role of breast feeding in family planning. *WHO Protein Advisory Group Bulletin* **5**(3), 5–10.

Rosenberg, Irwin H., Noel W. Solomons, and Douglas M. Levin (1976). Interaction of infection and nutrition: Some practical concerns. *Ecology of Food and Nutrition* **4**, 203–206.

Rosenbloom, L., and J. A. Sills (1975). Hypernatremic dehydration and infant mortality. *Archives of Diseases in Childhood* **50**, 750.

Ross, Constance A. C., and E. A. Dawes (1954). Resistance of the breast-fed infant to gastro-enteritis. *The Lancet* **1**(15 May), 994–998.

Rowland, Michael G. M., and Alison A. Paul (1981). Factors affecting lactation capacity: Implications for developing countries. In *Infant and Child Feeding*, edited by Jenny T. Bond, L. J. Filer, Jr., Gilbert A. Leveille, Angus M. Thomson, and William B. Weil, Jr. The Nutrition Foundation Monograph Series. Academic Press, New York, pp. 63–75.

Rowland, Michael G. M., R. A. E. Barrell, and Roger G. Whitehead (1978). Bacterial contamination in traditional Gambian weaning foods. *The Lancet* **1**(21 Jan.), 136–138.

Rowland, Michael G. M., T. J. Cole, and Roger G. Whitehead (1977). A quantitative study into the role of infection in determining nutritional status in Gambian children. *British Journal of Nutrition* **37**, 441–450.

Rowland, Thomas W., Roberto T. Zori, William R. Lafleur, and Edward O. Reiter (1982). Malnutrition and hypernatremic dehydration in breast-fed infants. *Journal of the American Medical Association* **247**, 1016–1017.

Royston, E. (1982). The prevalence of nutritional anemia in women in developing countries: A critical review of available information. *World Health Statistics Quarterly* **35**, 52–91.

Saarinen, Ulla M. (1978). Need for iron supplementation in infants on prolonged breast feeding. *Journal of Pediatrics* **93**(2), 177–180.

Saarinen, Ulla M., and Martti A. Siimes (1979). Role of prolonged breast feeding in infant growth. *Acta Paediatica Scandinavica* **68**, 245–250.

Salber, Eva J. (1956). Effect of different feeding schedules on growth of Bantu babies in the first week of life. *Journal of Tropical Pediatrics* **2**, 97–102.

Sanders, T. A. B., and D. J. Naismith (1979). A comparison of the influence of breast-feeding and bottle-feeding on the fatty acid composition of the erythrocytes. *British Journal of Nutrition* **41**, 619–623.

Sanders, T. A. B., M. Mistry, and D. J. Naismith (1984). The influence of a maternal diet rich in linoleic acid on brain and retinal docosahenxaenoic acid in the rat. *British Journal of Nutrition* **51**, 57–66.

Sandström, Brittmarie, Åke Cederblad, and Bo Lönnderdal (1983). Zinc absorption from human milk, cow's milk, and infant formulas. *American Journal of Diseases of Children* **137**, 726–729.

Sanguansermsri, J., P. György, and G. Zilliken (1974). Polyamines in human and cow's milk. *American Journal of Clinical Nutrition* **27**, 859–865.

Sauls, Henry S. (1979). Potential effect of demographic and other variables in studies comparing morbidity of breast-fed and bottle-fed infants. *Pediatrics* **64**, 523–527.

Saxton, George Albert, Jr., and D. M. Serwadda (1969). Human birth interval in East Africa. *Journal of Reproduction and Fertility*, suppl. 6, 83–88.

Schaefer, O. (1971). Otitis media and bottle-feeding. An epidemiological study of infant feeding habits and incidence of recurrent and chronic middle ear disease in Canadian Eskimos. *Canadian Journal of Public Health* **62**, 478–489.

Schallenberger, E., D. W. Richardson, and E. Knobil (1981). Role of prolactin in the lactational amenorrhea of the rhesus monkey (Macaca mulatta). *Biology of Reproduction* **25**, 370–374.

Schutz, Yves, Aaron Lechtig, and Robert B. Bradfield (1980). Energy expenditures and food intakes of lactating women in Guatemala. *American Journal of Clinical Nutrition* **33**, 892–902.

Scrimshaw, Nevin S., Carl E. Taylor, and John E. Gordon (1968). *Interactions of Nutrition and Infection*. World Health Organization Monograph Series no. 57. Geneva.

Seip, Martin, and Sverre Halvorsen (1956). Erythrocyte production and iron stores in premature infants during the first months of life. *Acta Paediatrica* **45**, 600–617.

Selner, J. C., D. A. Merrill, and H. N. Claman (1968). Salivary immunoglobulin and albumin:

Development during the newborn period. *Journal of Pediatrics* **72**, 685–689.

Seward, Jane F., and Mary K. Serdula (1984). Infant feeding and infant growth. *Pediatrics* **74**, 728–762.

Sharman, Albert (1951). Ovulation after pregnancy. *Fertility and Sterility* **2**, 371–393.

Shatrugna, Veena, Namala Raghuramula, and Krishnamurthy Prema (1982). Serum prolactin levels in undernourished Indian lactating women. *British Journal of Nutrition* **48**, 193–199.

Short, Roger V. (1983). The biological basis for the contraceptive effect of breast-feeding. In *Advances in International Maternal and Child Health*. Vol. 3, edited by Derrick B. Jelliffe and E. F. Patrice Jelliffe. Oxford University Press, Oxford, pp. 27–39.

Siimes, Martti A., Erkki Vuori, and Pekka Kuitunen (1971). Breast milk iron–A declining concentration during the course of lactation. *Acta Paediatrica Scandinavica* **68**, 29–31.

Silverstein, Arthur M., and Robert A. Prendergast (1964). Fetal response to antigenic stimulus. IV. Rejection of skin homografts by the fetal lamb. *Journal of Experimental Medicine* **119**, 955–964.

Simhon, Alberto, Robert H. Yolken, and Leonardo Mata (1979). S-IgA cholera toxin and rotavirus antibody in human colostrum. *Acta Paediatrica Scandinavica* **68**, 161–164.

Simpson, I. A., and A. Y. Chow (1956). The thiamine content of human milk in Malaya. Part I. The "normal" level of thiamine in milk from Malay, Chinese and Indian women. *Journal of Tropical Pediatrics* **2**, 3–17.

Simpson-Hebert, Mayling (1977). Breastfeeding in Iran and its relation to fertility. Ph.D. dissertation, University of North Carolina at Chapel Hill.

Simpson-Hebert, Mayling (1980). Breastfeeding and body contact. *Populi* **7**(2), 17–22.

Simpson-Hebert, Mayling, and Sandra L. Huffman (1981). The contraceptive effect of breastfeeding. *Studies in Family Planning* **12**, 125–133.

Sinclair, A. J., and M. A. Crawford (1972). The accumulation of arachidonate and docosahexaenoate in the developing rat brain. *Journal of Neurochemistry* **19**, 1753–1758.

Singarimbun, Masri, and Chris Manning (1976). Breastfeeding amenorrhea and abstinence in a Javanese village: A case study of Mojolama. *Studies in Family Planning* **7**, 175–179.

Smith, C. Wayne, and Arnold S. Goldman (1971). Macrophages from human colostrum. Multinucleated giant cell formation by phytohemagglutinin and concanavilin A. *Experimental Cell Research* **66**, 317–320.

Sosa, Roberto, Marshall Klaus, and Juan J. Urrutia (1976). Feed the nursing mother, thereby the infant. *Journal of Pediatrics* **88**, 668–670.

Stephens, Susan, C. R. Kennedy, P. K. Lakhani, and M. K. Brenner (1984). *In vivo* immune responses of breast- and bottle-fed infants to tetanus toxoid antigen and to normal gut flora. *Acta Paediatrica Scandinavica* **73**, 426–432.

Stiehm, E. Richard, and H. Hugh Fudenberg (1966). Serum levels of immune globulins in health and disease: A survey. *Pediatrics* **37**, 715–727.

Stites, Daniel P., and Charles S. Pavia (1979). Ontogeny of human T cells. *Pediatrics* **64**(suppl.), 795–801.

Sturman, John A., Gerald Gaull, and Neils C. R. Raiha (1970). Absence of cystathionase in human fetal liver: Is cystine essential? *Science* **169**(3 July), 74–76.

Sturman, John A., David K. Rassin, and Gerald E. Gaull (1977a). Minireview: Taurine in development. *Life Sciences* **21**, 1–22.

Sturman, John A., David K. Rassin, and Gerald E. Gaull (1977b). Taurine in developing rat brain: Transfer of [35S] taurine to pups via the milk. *Pediatric Research* **11**, 28–33.

Sullivan, John L., David W. Barry, Susan J. Lucas, and Paul Albrecht (1975). Measles infection of human mononuclear cells. I. Acute infection of peripheral blood lymphocytes and monocytes. *Journal of Experimental Medicine* **142**, 773–784.

Sundararaj, Regina, and Sheila M. Pereira (1975). Dietary intakes and food taboos of lactating women in a south Indian community. *Tropical and Geographical Medicine* **27**, 189–193.

Surjono, Dani, S. D. Ismadi, Suwardji, and Jon E. Rohde (1980). Bacterial contamination and dilution of milk in infant feeding bottles. *Journal of Tropical Pediatrics* **26**, 58–61.

Suzuki, S., Alan Lucas, Penny J. Lucas, and R. R. A. Coombs (1983). Immunoglobulin concentrations and bacterial antibody titres in breast-milk from mothers of "pre-term" and "term" infants. *Acta Paediatrica Scandinavica* **72**, 671–677.

Taggert, Nan R., Ruth M. Holliday, W. Z. Billiwicz, Frank E. Hytten, and Angus M. Thomson (1967). Changes in skinfolds during pregnancy. *British Journal of Nutrition* **21**, 439–451.

Taitz, L. S. (1971). Infantile overnutrition among artificially fed infants in the Sheffield region. *British Medical Journal* **1**(6 Feb.), 315–316.

Taylor, Brent, Jane Wadsworth, Jean Golding, and Neville Butler (1982). Breast-feeding, bronchitis, and admissions for lower respiratory illness and gastroenteritis during the first five years. *The Lancet* **1**(29 May), 1227–1229.

Thein, M. (1979). Study on milk vitamin A, serum vitamin A and serum protein levels of lactating mothers of Bochessa village, rural Ethiopia. *East African Medical Journal* **56**, 542–547.

Thomson, Angus M., W. Z. Billewicz, Barbara Thompson, and I. A. McGregor (1966). Body weight changes during pregnancy and lactation in rural African (Gambian) women. *Journal of Obstetrics and Gynaecology of the British Commonwealth* **73**, 724–733.

Thomson, Angus M., Frank E. Hytten, and W. Z. Billewicz (1970). The energy cost of human lactation. *British Journal of Nutrition* **24**, 565–572.

Tomasi, Thomas B., and John M. Beinenstock (1968). Secretory immunoglobulins. *Advances in Immunology* **9**, 1–96.

Totterdell, Barbara M., J. E. Banatvala, and I. L. Chrystie (1983). Studies on human lacteal rotavirus antibodies by immune electron microscopy. *Journal of Medical Virology* **11**, 167–175.

Totterdell, Barbara M., I. L. Chrystie, and J. E. Banatvala (1980). Cord blood and breast milk antibodies in neonatal rotavirus infection. *British Medical Journal* **280** (22 March), 828–836.

Tucker, H. Allen (1979). Endocrinology of lactation. *Seminars in Perinatology* **3**, 199–223.

Tyson, John E. (1977). Nursing and prolactin secretion: Principal determinants in the mediation of puerperal infertility. In *Prolactin and Human Reproduction*, edited by Pier Giorgio Crosignani and Claude Robyn. Proceedings of the Serono Symposia. Academic Press, New York.

Tyson, John E., John N. Carter, Barbara Andreassen, Janice Huth, and Beverly Smith (1978). Nursing-mediated prolactin and luteinizing hormone secretion during puerperal lactation. *Fertility and Sterility* **30**, 154–162.

Tyson, John E., R. S. Freedman, Alfredo Pérez, H. A. Zacur, and J. Zanartu (1976). Significance of the secretion of human prolaction and gonadotropin for puerperal lactational infertility. *Breast-feeding and the Mother*. Ciba Foundation Symposium, 45 (n.s.). Elsevier/Excerpta Medica/North-Holland, Amsterdam, pp. 49–71.

Ueda, Hiroshi, Akira Nakanishi, and Motohiko Ichijo (1980a). Immunochemical quantitation of serum complement components in SFD and AFD infants. *Tohoku Journal of Experimental Medicine* **132**, 111–116.

Ueda, Hiroshi, Akira Nakanishi, and Motohiko Ichijo (1980b). Immunoglobins in newborns, particularly in term SFD infants. *Tohoku Journal of Experimental Medicine* **132**, 31–35.

United Kingdom. Department of Health and Social Security (1980). *Present Day Practice in Infant Feeding: 1980. Report of a Working Party of the Panel on Child Nutrition, Committee on Medical Aspects of Food Policy.* Report on Health and Social Subjects no. 20. London.

The United Nations University. World Hunger Programme (1979). *Protein-Energy Requirements under Conditions Prevailing in Developing Countries: Current Knowledge and Research Needs. Food and Nutrition Bulletin* suppl. 1. WHTR-1/UNUP-18. [Tokyo].

Vahlquist, Bo (1958). The transfer of antibodies from mother to offspring. *Advances in Pediatrics* **10**, 305–338.

Valverde, Victor, Hernán L. Delgado, Elena Hurtado, and Robert E. Klein (1981). Maternal weight changes and energy intake during pregnancy and lactation. Paper presented to the XII International Congress of Nutrition, San Diego, California, 16–21 August.

Venkatchalam, P. S., T. P. Susheela, and Parvathi Rau (1967). Effect of nutritional supplementation during early infancy on growth of infants. *Journal of Tropical Pediatrics* **13**, 70–76.

Villa-Real, Romulo (1975). Breast-feeding in the Philippines. A benefit-cost analysis. School of Economics, University of the Philippines, Quezon City.

Viseshakul, Duangmanee (1976). Growth rate, feeding practices, and dietary intake of Thai infants under two years old in central Bangkok. *Journal of Human Nutrition* **30**, 71–78.

Viteri, Fernando E., and R. E. Schneider (1974). Gastrointestinal alterations in protein-calorie malnutrition. *Medical Clinics of North America* **58**(6), 1487–1505.

Vorherr, Helmuth (1974). *The Breast: Morphology and Lactation.* Academic Press, New York.

Vukavić, Tamara (1984). Timing of the gut closure. *Journal of Pediatric Gastroenterology and Nutrition* **3**, 700–703.

Walker, A. R. P., Barbara Richardson, and Faith Walker (1972). The influence of numerous pregnancies and lactation on bone dimensions in South African Bantu and Caucasian mothers. *Clinical Science* **42**, 189–196.

Walker, W. Allen (1979). Antigen penetration across the immature gut: Effect of immunologic and maturational factors in colostrum. In *Immunology of Breast Milk*, edited by Pearay L. Ogra and Delbert H. Dayton. A Monograph of the National Institute of Child Health and Human Development. Raven Press, New York, pp. 227–235.

Warren, Robert J., Martha L. Lepow, Glenn E. Bartsch, and Frederick C. Robbins (1961). The influence of breast milk on intestinal infection with Sabin type 1 poliovirus vaccine. *American Journal of Diseases of Children* **102**, 685–686.

Warren, Robert J., Martha S. Lepow, Glenn E. Bartsch, and Frederick C. Robbins (1964). The relationship of maternal antibody, breast-feeding, and age to the susceptibility of newborn infants to infection with attenuated poliovirus. *Pediatrics* **34**, 4–13.

Waterlow, J. C. (1981). Observations on the suckling's dilemma—A personal view. *Journal of Human Nutrition* **35**, 85–98.

Waterlow, J. C., and Angus M. Thomson (1979). Observations on the adequacy of breast-feeding. *The Lancet* **2**(4 Aug.), 238–242.

Waterlow, J. C., Ann Ashworth, and Mary Griffiths (1980). Faltering in infant growth in less-developed countries. *The Lancet* **2**(29 Nov.), 1176–1178.

Watson, M. A., E. S. Alford, C. W. Dill, R. L. Richter, and C. Garza (1982). Compositional changes during sequential sampling of human milk. *Nutrition Reports International* **26**, 1105–1111.

Weaver, Elizabeth A., Helen E. Rudloff, Randall M. Goldblum, Charles P. Davis, and Armond S. Goldman (1984). Secretion of immunoglobulin A by human milk leukocytes initiated by surface membrane stimuli. *Journal of Immunology* **132**, 684–689.

Welbourn, H. F. (1958). Bottle feeding: A problem of modern industrializing societies. *Journal of Tropical Pediatrics* **3**, 157–166.

Wellin, Edward (1955). Maternal and infant feeding practices in a Peruvian village. *Journal of the American Dietetic Association* **31**, 889–894.

Whitehead, Roger G. (1979). Nutrition and lactation. *Postgraduate Medical Journal* **55**, 303–310.

Whitehead, Roger G., ed. (1983). *Maternal Diet, Breast-Feeding Capacity, and Lactational Infertility. Report of a Joint UNU/WHO Workshop Held in Cambridge, United Kingdom, 9–11 March 1981.* WHTR-5/UNUP-338. The United Nations University, [Tokyo].

Whitehead, Roger G., and Alison A. Paul (1981). Infant growth and human milk requirements. A fresh approach. *The Lancet* **2**(25 July), 161–163.

Whitehead, Roger G., and Alison A. Paul (1984). Growth charts and the assessment of infant feeding practices in the Western world and in developing countries. *Early Human Development* **9**, 187–207.

Whitehead, Roger G., Alison A. Paul, and Michael G. M. Rowland (1980). Lactation in Cambridge and in the Gambia. In *Topics in Paediatrics*. Vol. 2. *Nutrition in Childhood*, edited by Brian Wharton. Pittman Medical, Turnbridge Wells, England, pp. 22–33.

Whitehead, Roger G., Michael G. M. Rowland, Melanie Hutton, Andrew M. Prentice, Elisabeth Müller, and Alison A. Paul (1978). Factors influencing lactation performance in rural Gambian mothers. *The Lancet* **2**(22 July), 178–181.

WHO. See also World Health Organization.

WHO/NRC Meeting (1983). Breast-feeding and fertility regulation: Current knowledge and programme policy implications. *Bulletin of the World Health Organization* **61**, 371–382.

Wickizer, Thomas M., and Lawrence B. Brilliant (1981). Testing for polychlorinated biphenyls in human milk. *Pediatrics* **68**, 411–415.

Widdowson, Elsie M. (1976). Changes in the body and its organs during lactation: Nutritional implications. In *Breast Feeding and the Mother*. Ciba Foundation Symposium 45 (n.s.). Elsevier/Excerpta Medica/North Holland, Amsterdam, pp. 103–118.

Widdowson, Elsie M., M. Joy Dauncey, D. M. T. Gairdner, J. H. P. Jonxis, and Marta Pelikan-Filipkova (1975). Body fat of British and Dutch infants. *British Medical Journal* **1**(22 Mar.), 653–655.

Williams, R. C., and R. J. Gibbons (1972). Inhibition of bacterial adherence by secretory immunoglobulin A: A mechanism of antigen disposal. *Science* **177**(25 Aug.), 697–699.

Wilson, John F., Douglas C. Heiner, and M. Eugene Lahey (1964). Milk-induced gastrointestinal bleeding in infants with hypochromic microcytic anemia. *Journal of the American Medical Association* **189**, 568–572.

Winberg, J., and G. Wessner (1971). Does breast milk protect against septicaemia in the newborn? *The Lancet* **1**(29 May), 1091–1094.

Wood, James, W. Daina Lai, Patricia L. Johnson, Kenneth L. Campbell, and Ila A. Maslar (forthcoming). Lactation and birth-spacing in highland New Guinea. *Journal of Biosocial Science*.

Woodbury, Robert M. (1922). The relation between breast and artificial feeding and infant mortality. *American Journal of Hygiene* **2**, 668–687.

Woolridge, M. W., T. V. How, R. F. Drewett, P. Rolfe, and J. David Baum (1982). The continuous measurement of milk intake at a feed in breast-fed babies. *Early Human Development* **6**, 365–373.

World Health Organization (1981). *Contemporary Patterns of Breast Feeding. Report on the WHO Collaborative Study on Breast-Feeding*. Geneva.

World Health Organization. Director General (1984). Infant and young child nutrition. (*Progress and Evaluation Report; Status of Implementation of the International Code of Marketing of Breast-milk Substitutes*.) 37th World Health Assembly. Provisional agenda item 20. A37/6. Geneva.

World Health Organization. Division of Family Health (1980). The incidence of low birth weight: A critical review of available information. *World Health Statistics Quarterly* **33**, 197–224.

World Health Organization and Food and Agriculture Organization. Ad Hoc Expert Committee (1973). *Energy and Protein Requirements. Report of a Joint FAO/WHO Ad Hoc Expert Committee.* World Health Organization Technical Report Series no. 522. FAO Nutrition Meetings Report Series no. 52. Geneva.

Worthington-Roberts, Bonnie S., Joyce Vermeersch, and Sue Rodwell Williams (1985). *Nutrition in Pregnancy and Lactation.* 3d ed. Times Mirror/Mosby, St. Louis.

Wray, Joe D., and Alfredo Aguirre (1969). Protein-calorie malnutrition in Candelaria, Colombia. I. Prevalence; Social and demographic causal factors. *Journal of Tropical Pediatrics* **15**, 76–98.

Yap, P. L., A. Pryde, P. J. Latham, and D. B. L. McLelland (1979). Serum IgA in the neonate. Molecular size, concentration and effect of breast feeding. *Acta Paediatrica Scandinavica* **68**, 695–700.

Yekutiel, Perez, Eric Peritz, and Joseph Mandil (1958). A field study of infantile diarrhoea in Israel. *Journal of Tropical Pediatrics* **3**, 175–183.

Young, Charlotte M., Gladys C. Hagan, Ruth E. Tucker, and Walter D. Foster (1952). A comparison of dietary study methods. II. Dietary history vs. seven-day record vs. 24-hr. recall. *Journal of the American Dietetic Association* **28**, 218–221.

Zeitlin, Marian F., Z. Masangkay, M. Consolacion, and M. Nass (1978). Breast feeding and nutritional status in depressed urban areas of greater Manila, Phillipines. *Ecology of Food and Nutrition* **7**, 103–113.

Zeitlin, Marian F., Nina P. Schlossman, Michael J. Newar, Joe D. Wray, and John B. Stanbury (1980). *Nutrition-Fertility Interactions in Developing Countries: Implications for Program Design.* Prepared under the auspices of the Massachusetts Institute of Technology International Nutrition and International Population Initiative Programs and Abt Associates, Inc., Cambridge, Mass., for the Office of Policy Development and Program Review, Agency for International Development under contract #AID/otr. 147-179-132.

NAME INDEX

SUBJECT INDEX